Things Are Working Out
How Fitness Shaped My First 50 Years

Lisa Safran

For Dad

You can.

Push through this feeling right now.

Be comfortable with uncomfortable.

Dig a little deeper because you want this.

Honor the chaos in your head.
Welcome it into the room, and then escort it out the door.

Be stronger than you think.

PROLOGUE

They used to call me "HercuLisa."

It all started in March 1966, when the name "Lisa" was trending, and I was making my entrance into the world at Booth Memorial Hospital in Queens, New York. I came in at a whopping nine pounds, one ounce. No scrawny chicken legs for me—I was a Butterball turkey from the start. My dad, Mr. Dry Wit and Creativity, coined my nickname. It was the perfect combination of the popular 1960s' girl's name and Hercules, the mythological Greek god who was known for his strength and power.

My dad was enamored with muscles. Growing up, I would watch him refer to his little black notebook, a six-ring binder about the size of a small paperback novel, for exercises and workouts to sculpt his muscles like those of pioneering bodybuilders such as John Grimek and Reg Park. After dinner sometimes or on a rainy Saturday afternoon, Dad would exercise in his bedroom, one of two bedrooms in our tiny Queens apartment, and I would watch. There would be old, rusty weights and dumbbells strewn across the carpeted floor. Rust streaks stained his sweat-soaked undershirts as he clanked the weights around while watching the small black-and-white TV with the aluminum-foiled rabbit ears. Pushing, pulling, pressing, raising these iron blocks over his head. I had no idea what he was doing, but it was fascinating to watch.

There was a miniature statue of Michelangelo's *David* on Dad's dresser. About as tall as one of my baby dolls, *David* always seemed to be watching, too. Perched on a black marble pedestal, *David* was chiseled out of white stone, with rippling abdominal muscles and sweeping thighs that went far beyond his kneecaps. It was a stark difference to my dad's physique, which reminded me of one of my storybook characters: Humpty Dumpty. Like Humpty, Dad had an enormous belly, with long stick legs and arms. When I would hug him, I would squeeze extra tight to try to make my hands connect behind his back.

Dad's father, Grandpa Dick, was built exactly the same way. We would visit Grandpa and Grandma every summer in Florida where family antics would ensue. The 8mm sprocket films captured Dad and Grandpa barefoot in the sunny backyard, deep in the coarse grass, performing belly bumps in their sleeveless ribbed undershirts and long polyester shorts. Grandpa's shirt pulled tightly across his tummy, making the shirt sheer enough to see his sinkhole belly button. "HercuLisa!" Dad and Grandpa would call me over and I would join them in making funny faces to the camera, pretending like I was wedged in between a jumbo belly sandwich.

I liked having a nickname that was mine and only mine, and a family silly enough to give it to me. It stuck with me for many years, until I developed an awareness that people were looking at me funny when Dad would call me HercuLisa in public. *What kind of a girl's nickname is that?* I could see the judgment in people's eyes. In time, HercuLisa fizzled out to an occasional, hey-remember-when-we-used-to-call-you reference. I was more than happy to keep it our family secret.

It would take many years before I would feel strong enough to say the name out loud to someone in conversation. In fact, I felt proud because, by that point, I finally understood what being HercuLisa meant to me.

THE SNACK TABLE ERA

I grew up on TV dinners and TV. It was the 1970s, and we had an enormous for the time 25-inch console television in the living room; it was the design focal point in which all elements revolved around. Lazy-Boy recliners and snack tables arched around it, creating a theater-like vibe before in-home entertainment rooms ever existed. The heavy, sienna-colored drapes would get drawn throughout the day to avoid the annoying glare on the screen, so the room was always darker than the day. And then there was the remote. Tiny, cool metal box with three buttons—yes, three. Channel, volume, and an on/off in the brightest orange in case your eye couldn't discern the point of power from the others. This nifty device would flip me through a limited supply of channels (2, 4, 5, 7, 9, 11, and 13), but the thrill was in the click. Sometimes, when I changed from station to station, I'd zone out to the split-second sliver of wavy darkness in between channels.

I spent hours a short distance from a boob tube that fed my mind with politically incorrect shows including *All in the Family*, way too sexy for my age soap operas like *All My Children*, violent bunny cartoons with exploding bombs from the Acme Company, and after-school specials about kids trapped in dire situations. *Bad Ronald* was the story of a teenage boy who accidentally kills a girl who was bullying him. His mom hides him in a secret compartment behind the walls of his home to avoid the police, but then she dies, and the house gets sold to another family with Ronald still stuck behind the Sheetrock. It was perfect, wholesome after-school TV for a preteen to be watching alone after a long day of academia.

There was enough real-life bullying to make the story hit home for me. Jody, a girl in my second-grade class, was intrigued with my origami skills. My best friend, Mayumi, had taught me how to make a simple pouch and a balloon. The pouch was quite handy for storing an eraser or a paper clip or two. Jody caught a glimpse of my paper-folding skills and threatened me to make her 50 pouches by the next school day *or else*. I had no idea what *or else* meant; I just sensed that Jody meant business and that I had better get folding. There were no anti-bullying movements to get the bullies to stop or to empower the bullied. The picked-on suffered in silence. After school, in an attempt to console the hurt, we ate Count Chocula breakfast cereal straight from the box while watching *Popeye*. He was always feasting on canned spinach, which looked disgusting, but he did have the most powerful-looking arms I had ever seen. Popeye may have been all sweet and kind before downing a can of spinach, but if you messed with him like Jody did with me, he'd knock you out.

Facing our outstanding TV was a collapsible snack table with a picture of a beautiful French countryside printed on the metal tray. It was colorful enough to camouflage ketchup plops from my tator tots and crumb breakaways from my Entenmann's coffee cake.

Behind the sturdy snack table, in front of the behemoth television, was me. Young HercuLisa. Still naturally on the slightly plumper side, but nothing so remarkable to get someone to scream at me to get off the sofa and order a set of workout CDs. Then again, it was the '70s. There were no workout CDs. To *work out* meant you were doing a hard math problem at school or something fortunate happened. *That situation really worked out.*

We were all couch potatoes. The etymology of the phrase "couch potato" had first appeared in print in the late 1970s, but I was pioneering the idiom before it was even a real thing. Fitness just wasn't in the vocabulary. Without an ounce of guilt or a parental nag to "turn that thing off and get up!" was me, the TV, a snack table, and an edible goodie that came wrapped in plastic or in a box. Other than in the cartoon *Fat Albert*, the word "fat" wasn't relevant in my daily vernacular. I loved Fat Albert—he was funny and kind, and he shuffled across my TV screen trying to catch his friends as well as his breath. Dad had a shape like Albert's, but it was all just a matter of fact to me, not fat.

Except for an occasional boy-chasing-girl sprint in the schoolyard, I embodied inactivity. My maternal grandmother loved my juicy cheeks and would pinch them daily. I dressed in bell-bottom jeans, striped acrylic sweaters (with stripes running the unflattering horizontal way), and Puma Clyde sneakers. I loved my blue suede Puma Clydes more than anything else in my closet. I loved saying the name: Puma Clyde. I would take my time and let the Clyde glide. My Puma Clydes made me feel cool in ways I had never experienced before. I felt, well, sporty. The suede was dreamy and creamy, just like a Devil Dog, where spongy chocolate cake meets white artificial cream. My mom brought me to the neighborhood shoe store where the salesman sat on a small, triangular stool and placed my foot into the metal measuring contraption. I endured the cold shock from the metal coming through my thin sock knowing that new shoes were coming. Clyde cost a bazillion dollars, but Mom knew how much I wanted them and, because I didn't ask for much, they were mine. I wore them home from the store and I rarely took them off.

Technically, these were my first pair of real sneakers. I wore them with no intention of doing anything else but exercising my right to take them off and sit on the couch after school. Prior to these, I had the cheaper, generic version of Keds. We called them "skips," a name that couldn't have been more indicative of my lackadaisical physical effort. These sneakers had a thin fabric upper and were completely unsupportive. My older sister, Sharon, wore skips, too. My parents didn't own sneakers. Dad had Hush Puppies, which were his casual wear loafers. Mom only wore heels, whether they were snazzy platform sandals or super-high, skinny-heeled boots. She was the mom who was always decked out in groovy bell-bottom pants and a flowy top, and she never left the house without lipstick. I thought she was the most beautiful woman in the world.

We were not the family that would bike to the park or swim at a lake. We didn't play volleyball or tennis. But we did walk everywhere. It was inherent in city living. Dad walked to and from work each day at his dental office on Parsons Boulevard in Flushing, a good mile from home. My sister and I walked to and from school. Mom hoofed it in heels whether she was walking with us to school or running errands down Main Street.

We may have been physically inactive, but we were anything but lazy. Hard work was one of the hallmarks of our family values. It manifested in our approach to everything we did, from the way my mom meticulously tended to the family to my father's work in his dental practice. It also came through in their expectations of how we applied ourselves at school, as well as our integrity and honesty as people. We were an earnest bunch. We poured ourselves into things we were passionate about. I was fiercely dedicated to my school work. My sister and I played Barbies like nobody's business. My mom transferred all of her dedication as a school teacher to be a stay-at-home mom. My dad immersed himself in researching topics of interest, from innovations in dentistry to techniques in bodybuilding. Bodybuilding was a hobby of his and he studied it at the library, reading up on anatomy and kinesiology, always in search of new exercises to add to his little black book. In addition to his work as a dentist, he was an inventor with multiple patents. We were a worker-bee kind of crowd.

But, yes, we did our share of loafing around. If you worked hard all day, you had every right to soak in an after-school special, a cheesy soap opera, or an episode of the scandalous *Dynasty* on prime-time TV. Without even striving for it, we had balance in our daily lives. We walked everywhere, got up and down from desks, took staircases because the elevator was often broken in our apartment building, and walked to the grocery store pushing a shopping cart that later came back weighted with a hefty load of food. Living in the city and not owning a car made movement a necessity.

My only formalized activity exception was Wednesday, from 4 to 5 pm. Wednesdays were the "big move" day for me as I strolled to the Brooklyn Conservatory (in Queens—go figure) just one block down and one over from my apartment building. This tiny building, surrounded by prewar buildings, was where I took ballet once a week for seven years. On my mini stroll over, with my faux patent leather, box-shaped dance bag slung over my shoulder, I imagined myself being a professional dancer one day. The dance bag had a secret slim compartment for shoes (I learned how to layer the shoes, one upside down against the other, for them to fit) and a leaping dancer's silhouette on the side. If only my legs would leap that high. I always wore my leotard and tights under my street clothes. The seam of the tights pressing up against my toes inside my Clydes usually hurt, but the walk was short enough to endure.

Ms. Hauser taught me how to be a ballerina. She was taller than most of the dads I had ever seen, and with a soft but powerful voice and accent that made it hard to understand her direction sometimes. I followed her hands and body language instead. She was a graceful dancer and a patient teacher. When she'd demonstrate a pirouette, her entire body would fill the room. When she played the piano for us, her hands became tarantulas claiming territory. When she shouted directives over the sound of the record player spinning Tchaikovsky, she was a drill sergeant. When she hugged me after I mastered a turn without toppling over, she was a weighted velvet princess cape over my proud shoulders. Ms. Hauser applauded my hard-earned fifth position and the angle of my right foot against the left. Her smile told me that my hard work was paying off. She made me feel like the most beautiful ballerina in all of Flushing.

I had two ballerina outfits that I alternated for each class: black leotard with pale pink tights, and the antithesis, pale pink leotard with black tights. I squeezed myself into the spandex every Wednesday after school and hurried off to class. Never once did I pause to examine how these outfits looked on me. It was all about how I felt in them. And I felt excited, eager, beautiful, and graceful—until the day Patty started counting.

Patty was a girl in my ballet class. She was as slight as a twig with a black pouf of short, curly hair. She looked like a dirty Q-tip. Her hands and feet reminded me of Barbie's, so tiny and delicate I could snap them off if I were mad enough. Patty's black leotard hung around her flat-as-a-pancake bottom, while mine wedged up my ample rump. Her cap sleeves sat loosely around the top part of her arms, while mine clung like Popeye's sailor T-shirt. I noticed these things like the way a painter sees shapes and color, but it was all in the category of curious observations. None of it was attached to judgment of others or me. Then, one day, while clad in my pink leo, Patty pointed her microscopic finger at my tummy. "One, two, three, four rolls of fat!" she announced. The other girls laughed. *Swan Lake* swirled in my ears, along with Ms. Hauser's deep voice syncing with her rhythmic hand claps, and Patty found her place in the line just in time to spin across the room. I was nine or ten years old, in a little room with mirrors everywhere. People were looking at me and laughing. I was looking at myself and holding back the tears. *I'm fat?*

My mother picked me up after class with her bright pink lips, beaming at me like always. The fox fur collar of her winter coat cradled her neck like a movie star's. But I didn't feel like smiling back. Patty had triggered something in me. It made me look at other people, particularly females, with a more critical eye. Poof, just like that, in one simple dance class, the perception of my body image had changed.

Who else is fat? Is Mom fat? What exactly is fat? I guess Grandpa is fat, so Daddy is fat, too. But what about me? I couldn't get the dialogue in my head to quiet down. My father's stomach was enormous. My mother jokingly called it "the corporation" as if it had a force of its own. I had always thought of Daddy like a big, cuddly teddy bear. He probably weighed around 250 pounds, which, in time I would learn, was way too much for his 5'10" frame. I never saw him any other way but this size. It just was the way he was.

This fresh encounter with Patty had me noticing the loose, blubbery arms that my grandmother threw around me every day when I came home from school and visited her in the office of our apartment building. (She was the manager of the building.) *Was that fat?* It just felt like love up until then. My glamorous, always decked-out mother had a pouch of squishy flesh right below her belly button. *Was that fat?* Mom's skin was soft and pale, and her tummy was like a mushy pillow I could rest on when a fever made my head hurt. She had a little scar on the right side of her tummy where she said a doctor cut her during an emergency appendectomy when she was 20 years old. Suddenly, I was looking at everyone, especially other girls, with a critical adipose lens. Conversely, this made me notice girls who were the opposite of fat. *Skinny.* I was still close enough to the generation that grew up with Twiggy, the super-thin model, to know who she was. I had lots of Barbies, with their cinched waists, big boobies, and major thigh gaps. The magazines I read had pictures of girls whose bodies looked nothing like mine.

There were girls at school with arms so thin you could see muscle striations under their skin, and their legs were so twiggy that the knee bones would pop out. Nothing gathering underneath their clothing that people like Patty could count. At pick up after school, I would notice that their moms wore polyester slacks that clung to long, bony legs. My thighs rubbed together, and in the summer when sweat built up from the friction, I'd develop a rash. Old grandmas had thighs that rubbed together and arms that jiggled when they'd wave—not young girls like me. Young girls were supposed to be skinny and smooth, with spaces between body parts and bones you could see.

Maybe this self-perception was destined to happen. I was a 1970s' preteen, at the age where I was beginning to relate to my own body in ways I hadn't before. The outer me I was packaged in was not good enough. I was too much this, or not enough that. I couldn't shake the feeling. I also didn't know what to do with it. I walked around with a knot in my stomach all the time that found its way into cuticle picking. I began to dread going to dance class and having to be in my leotard in front of the other girls. I stopped wearing the slightly sheer pink one and only opted for the black; black was the color that the magazines said was slimming.

I tried to deal with the Pattys in my life by firing quips back at them. "Well, at least I'm not short!" and "Did you take your ugly pills today?" (The first one was mine; the latter was Mom's). But I was not really a quip kind of kid. Inside, the dialogue was more like, *Why are you making fun of me? Why are you making me want to cry?*

Still, I stuck with dance. I tried to focus on my hands and the way I could hold them in the perfect, delicate dancer position. It amazed me how slim and sinewy my hands could look even if I had one, two, three, four rolls of belly fat. Through dance, I was growing more and more aware of my preteen body but focusing on the parts I didn't like, finding it harder to put my attention toward my green eyes or the dimples that emerged when I smiled. Parts of my body were suddenly budding in different ways. Too big, too small, too this, too that. I secretly began to come up with other words to describe my shape—flub, flubby, flubber (I was reading Judy Blume's novel, *Blubber*), jiggly, wiggly, roly-poly, thunder thighs, just to name a few. The inner dialogue stuck in my head and occasionally made its way to a diary that came with a lock and key, but even that didn't feel like a safe place for my thoughts.

Eventually, my once-per-week ballet lessons progressed to dancing *en pointe*. All I ever wanted was to dance in those beautiful pointe shoes and feel like Cinderella in her glass slippers. They were elegant, pale pink, satin shoes with matching ribbons that I learned to crisscross up my anything-but-slender ankles. I learned how to wrap the puffy lamb's wool around my toes before entering these princess-like slippers to help in cushioning my toes. These shoes made me feel like Barbie, perpetually *en pointe*, and I didn't care that it felt like I was balancing my toes against a block of concrete. "Beauty is pain," I picked up from a magazine article. I would endure.

But the preteen years are a precarious time to be standing on your toes in a room surrounded by mirrors and judgmental little girls. As much as I loved to dance, and as much as I was excited to perform *Swan Lake en pointe* in a recital one day, I couldn't get past all the negativity and doubt and confusion inside of me. It was all so jumbled up inside my head and tummy. The only way out was to quit. My parents had the "Are you sure?" conversations with me, but in true, supportive fashion, they didn't push.

My single source of formal exercise for my entire childhood had come to a halt. All I had left was walking to and from school, walking to Main Street for shopping, going up and down the stairs of my apartment building, and occasionally running home from school on days when the threat of bullies throwing Nair hair removal at your head was looming. (This was usually just on Halloween, but the bullies were unpredictable.) Occasionally, my sister and I would pop on a record album and dance our hearts out in the living room. "The Locomotion" was a top hit for shaking our groove things. We'd dance so hard that our long, Marcia Brady type hair would cling to our necks and foreheads with sweat.

The only other mandatory exercise I had left was gym at school. None of my friends played a sport. There were a handful of gymnasts and the rare girl who threw a ball like a boy or played softball in a league that you had to drive to Long Island for, which could have been Italy when you're a kid from Flushing whose parents don't have a car. I was the girl who got picked last when divvying up teams. I was the one who couldn't dodge a dodge ball. Sometimes we played tag or jump rope or hopscotch if we could wrangle up a nub of chalk and a few willing bodies that weren't worried about looking uncool, but usually we sat around and ate snacks smuggled in from the corner deli. Processed cakes wrapped in cellophane with the beautiful Hostess logo with the heart on top. The heart equaled love. Twinkies, Ding Dongs, Fruit Pies, Ho Hos, Snow Balls, Suzy Q's, and the simply-named Cup Cakes with the fondant-like chocolate frosting and heavy, white frosting squiggle on top, and burst of white cream inside. I loved the squiggle. I would peel it off in one piece and save it to eat last. Each bite offered an instant burst of sugar followed by a thick cream-based center that made my teeth hurt.

We'd change into gym clothes to give the illusion of effort. It was the decade of solid-colored gym shorts with white piping and knee-high tube socks with double stripes around the calves. Tops were plain, solid colors or a rock concert T-shirt if you had an older sibling who somehow got to Jones Beach Theater from Queens (not an easy task unless you had a car; most families did not) to see AC/DC or Pink Floyd. Me, I could have been wearing a silk blouse. No sweat happening in my pits. We went outside, whether it was boiling hot or freezing cold, to play kick ball, dodge ball, or catch. In the winter, I kept my bouclé cowl neck sweater on to keep half warm. The outfit matched my effort. *Meh.* None of it excited me. The most interesting part was making sure that I looked halfway decent as I ran (and I say that word lightly) the bases, never making it to first base before the ball. I was neither an athlete nor athletic. I was the girl who threw like a girl, who practically skipped from base to base, who achieved the bare minimum scores on the physical fitness tests that the school was required to give the students each year. There was one girl who could do the pull-up hang for minutes at a time! Me, I jumped up to the position on the bar and, like a pile of snow thawing off the roof, just slid right down. There were the sit-ups, which I could do, but at a snail's pace and with lots of neck-cranking cheats along the way.

I didn't care if the other kids were faster or stronger. I just wanted to do my thing, and that included drawing and writing and daydreaming out a window. Put me in a room for hours with arts and crafts materials, magic markers, and a sketch book, and I would create a magical world that I wanted to crawl into. I didn't have an ounce of competitiveness in me. The only time I recall competing as a child was when I was chosen to represent my school in the Halloween Art Contest at a bank. It was me against 10 other kids from other local elementary schools.

Locked away with markers, a blank piece of oversized construction paper, and my imagination, I pondered the challenge: create your best Halloween picture. For the first time, the knot I had been carrying around in my tummy felt different. It was still there but I was feeling something good inside, too—exhilarated, nervous, giddy beyond belief. *Is this what competition feels like?* I quickly got lost in my work. I still remember my picture: an outdoor scene that included every Halloween icon imaginable. A witch on a broom, tombstones, ghosts, silhouettes of black cats, pumpkins—all integrated into some imagined landscape. When time was up, the artists were asked to leave the room for the judges to evaluate the work. After a short break over cookies and juice, the students were brought back in.

There were ribbons tacked onto all the pictures: gold, red, blue. From afar, I could see a black one on mine. *Black must be a consolation prize*, I thought. But when I got close enough to read the gold lettering, I was shocked to see First Prize. I won! I had never won anything before in my life. Someone at the bank took a picture of me holding my artwork and another banker person shaking my hand. The picture appeared in the local newspaper along with a short news story. Did I care about the $25 account that the bank started for me? Not really. All I cared about was the silky black ribbon with the gold embossed letters that proved I was a winner. It didn't matter how many rolls of fat I had—I was deemed the best at something and I had the silk ribbon to prove it. Yes, black was indeed very slimming.

My brush with competition ignited something inside of me that I hadn't paid any attention to. I always had a bit of the ham gene in me, having entered talent shows and signing up for parts in school plays. I sang "California, Here I Come" in an elementary school musical. I offered to play the piano part, too, and the teacher was elated. The problem was that I didn't really know how to play the piano; I only knew "Chopsticks." Dad, who was a proficient musician and played the accordion magnificently since he was a little boy, was giving me lessons at home on our electric organ. Why I thought, with a week or two of practice, I could pull it off in a school musical is completely beyond comprehension. A voice inside of me said *You can do this* when, in this particular situation, I really had no right to feel that way. The belief in self was admirable; the reality check, humbling.

Dad practiced with me for hours after school for a solid week. I was making progress, but I was beginning to realize that I was going to make a fool of myself, make my teacher mad and quite possibly, ruin the entire play. I eventually backed out, still with enough time for the teacher to play the piano instead, and I only did the singing part. However, this experience opened my eyes to the fact that I truly, honestly believed in myself, even when maybe I had no right to. My one, two, three, four rolls of tummy fat didn't matter when it came to the proficiency of my hands. Sketching out an imagined scene, attempting to navigate the piano keys, I thought I could do anything. I could visualize myself doing the unthinkable. My imagination was vivid.

While most of my childhood was filled with limited, noncompetitive activities, summertime was ripe with adventure. It was the time when accidental exercise was in full swing. We got off our bums to move, and not because it was good for us, or an adult was yelling at us to stop being couch potatoes, or the newspapers were scaring us with health statistics, but because it was fun. Being in an apartment all day during the sweltering summer heat, with only one air conditioner in my parent's bedroom that went on only at night, and the other in the living room that went on only if temperatures hit 1,000 degrees, was stifling.

My sister and I would go outside for hours, which is what kids who grew up in the city did. There was a park across the street and it was where we buckled up our jelly shoes to run around the public sprinklers, which seemed to be on all the time without any regard to water restrictions. The metallic smell of water gushed from the silver nozzle heads like a rain shower doused in chemicals. The stench of wet rubber shoes overpowered the smell of fruity beverages sipped from wilting, waxy paper cups. When I'd try to run from spout to spout, my legs felt like lead as the sopping jellies suctioned my feet to the concrete.

The alleyway behind my building was where we'd play handball against the brick wall until our palms burned. We'd sprint when we heard the bells from the Mr. Softee ice cream truck coming up the street. I couldn't lick the ears of my Black Cat cone fast enough to keep the soft serve from dripping down my arm. But my most favorite place of all for accidental exercise was Skyline Swim Club.

Skyline Swim Club was a private pool that was part of the fancy sky-rise building down the street. If you lived in Skyline, in one of those beautiful apartments with the terraces that were high enough to wave to the passengers in the planes leaving LaGuardia Airport, the pool access was free. Anyone else in the neighborhood could join for a fee for the summer or pay for a daily pass. Most families opted for the free sprinklers at the park. There were also the cigarette-smoking, sit-on-the-hoods-of-parked-cars kids who hopped the fence at night to sneak into another private pool next door at a building called The Newport. Not quite as fancy as Skyline, yet not as plain Jane as my building (which didn't have a name or a pool), The Newport had a pool with a diving board! The building also had a swanky lobby with cushioned furniture, and a few extra floors beyond the typical six to underscore, quite literally, higher status. Somehow, our modest lifestyle turned posh each summer as we enjoyed a family membership to Skyline Swim Club. It was the ultimate "fun in the sun" just like Barbie was always up for.

My father made the connection to exercise years before I was even born. I could see it every time he pulled out his clunky black weights and dumbbells, and little black notebook with strongman exercises categorized by body part. The equipment looked like torture chamber devices from the Middle Ages. He'd strap on archaic, weighted shoes and do leg raises off the edge of his bed. The heavy black straps anchored the weighted mechanisms to his bedroom slippers. He'd sit, with the little TV on for background noise, and curl dumbbells in his hands. He'd lay on the bed and press a thin metal bar with clanking weights on the ends off his chest. I'd come visit him, usually with a peanut butter and jelly sandwich in hand, while he was working out. His voice was breathy from effort and we'd converse. I'd watch the sweat pour off his face. Everything he was doing looked painful and not much fun, but it also intrigued me. There was always something so serious in his eyes when he exercised.

I wondered what exactly it was that he liked about all this. "What's this one for?" I'd ask repeatedly while flipping through the notebook, looking at his notes and diagrams. "Who's that?" I pointed to the black-and-white photo of a young man in a bathing suit. The man's muscles popped out like the *David* statue in my parents' room. His ribs stuck out, too, as if he had sucked in his entire stomach to take the picture. Dad looked at the picture and made that face he'd make after eating an entire bag of cookies before anyone else had a single one. "That's you, Daddy?" *When did the man in the picture turn into my dad?*

Dad seemed excited that someone in the family had taken an interest in his love for exercise. He taught me about Eugen Sandow, a bodybuilding pioneer born in the late 1800s who would eventually be dubbed "the father of modern bodybuilding." Dad showed me a quote from Sandow that read, "Nothing, in my opinion, is better than the use of the dumbbell for developing the whole system." I learned that strongmen, like Sandow, were viewed as exhibitionists who could perform tricks of strength to entertain the crowd, such as lifting a super-heavy dumbbell with one hand over their heads. In the 1930s, bodybuilding was shifting away from where strength was the only thing that impressed the crowd. People would now *ooh* and *aah* over the aesthetics of the muscles. Pretty soon, modern bodybuilding was taking off, with the arrival of the first competition, Mr. America. Bodybuilding skyrocketed in popularity for the next few decades. This brought fame to men like John Grimek, Steve Reeves, and Reg Park.

My father's exposure to these "gods" started in his teens when he began working out. He'd save up money to buy the muscle magazines that were filled with photos and exercises. The weights he used were primitive, but they were just enough to start building his muscles. When he attended college and then dental school, there was less time for exercise. And then he got married, started a dental practice, had my sister, got sick for a little bit and couldn't do much physical activity, and then had me. There was a whole other person under his belly that I didn't know anything about. Knowing that Dad kept returning to his "weight room" to reconnect with the guy in the black book made me want to get to know him, too.

Dad was an emotional eater. He'd teeter between claiming self-control through exercise and losing it through food. He would exercise when he was happy and eat when he was sad or frustrated. One activity fed the other. Always wrestling with what he looked like and what he imagined he could be, Dad's attempts at exercise were always two steps forward, one step back.

His eating was closely tied to habits, too. There was the food in front of the TV to accompany favorite shows like *Abbott and Costello* and *Chiller Theater*: chips, cookies, anything that came in a bag. Sunday meals at our favorite diner came with Dad's regular order of the Burger Deluxe, which was two cheeseburgers on two buns with double fries and onion rings. Dad would sprinkle salt on like the little girl from *The Partridge Family* shaking her tambourine. Mom would find candy wrappers in his coat pocket at the end of the day. He often took a small detour to stop into the candy store to pick up a *New York Times*, *Daily News,* and a Chunky candy bar.

Dad cycled from frustrated bouts in the kitchen to methodical attempts in his quasi-weight room. With the TV on and weights scattered across the room, he would work out. The workouts were always so precise, like he knew exactly what he was doing and *this time* it would be the start of something better. Like "I'll start again on Monday," over and over again. He kept notes to chart his progress. Reps, weights, exercises. But never, ever did he hop on the scale, which was hidden under the dresser.

Watching my father struggle brought both clarity and confusion to my own questioning and self-discovery. He was the greatest guy on the planet, so being like him was all I wanted to do. Yet, there was a struggle I couldn't fully understand or see, and that was scary. He would sit in his TV chair for hours listening to opera music. With eyes closed, tears would stream down his cheeks as Puccini's *La Bohéme* filled the room. *Why was he crying? What was he feeling? What was I feeling?* It was all so muddled up.

My dad's younger brother, Steve, on the other hand, was a physical Adonis. Uncle Steve epitomized good health; he had muscles on top of muscles, a strong jawline, thick black hair, and piercing green eyes. He worked out religiously and could do flips and handstands like a circus performer. He ate clean and embraced organic before it was even a movement. Fresh fruits and vegetables, juices and extracts, vitamins no one ever heard of. He eventually went vegan and studied Buddhism after living in India with his equally crunchy wife, my aunt Ladene, during their time together in the Peace Corps. No one expected him to be the one to die from leukemia at the age of 39. I was seven or eight years old when we went to visit him for the last time. He was sitting in his living room in lotus pose looking like the bendy flamingo statue on his front lawn in

Pompano Beach, Florida. Skinny, skinny legs. All head and torso. No muscle. The light in his green eyes still flickering until the very end.

So, growing up, I had this odd, unofficial, quasi-unhealthy exposure to exercise and fitness. There wasn't a right or wrong way to approach it, but it usually included seeing others caught in a struggle. Some battle between the body, which I could see, and some invisible force on the inside.

My first 15 years of life subjected me to admiration for the perfect physique, to goals unachieved, to being judged by others, to feelings I had no idea how to deal with, to believing in yourself, to never giving up, to the word *fat*. I grew up watching Dad struggle to reach a version of himself that he could calculate in notebooks but, in real life, could never make happen.

When he gave me my own set of dumbbells for my sixteenth birthday, a sleek pair of plastic, gold-colored five-pound weights, I knew that Dad was passing the torch.

THE IN-BETWEEN YEARS

My friends were getting gold jewelry and having fancy parties with DJs for their Sweet 16's. I got my first real leather purse. Very 1980s: white, puffy, and pleated with a gaudy flower on the front and a thin spaghetti strap. I also got gold but mine was plastic and weighty. The dumbbells. Beyond being a symbol of the special time Dad spent teaching me about exercise, the dumbbells were representative of a tool for my future. Dad was big on symbolic gifts, and he was able to make all kinds of statements about these dumbbells "building me up" and "shaping my future and my strength." I listened, but I secretly wished for a party.

I was 16 and, more than ever, I saw my physical self unlike the girls in my *Tiger Beat* magazines. They wore tight Jordache jeans that hugged their baby-sized butts. Their thigh gaps were wide enough to wave to someone on the other side. And they were always laughing. Toothy, white smiles so cheesy you could serve them with crackers. Everyone looked so skinny and so happy.

A Farrah Fawcett poster was taped to my bedroom wall. Farrah was an actress in *Charlie's Angels*, a show about a trio of women who solve crimes under the leadership of Charlie, a man we never see. He is simply piped in via speakers or phone calls. Typical 1980s' programming where the women are only as good as the men who tell them what to do. The three angels were stereotypical of the time—one a gorgeous, sophisticated, vixen brunette; one a normal, attractive brunette who was portrayed as the brains of the group, the egghead; and the sexy, sometimes ditzy blond, Farrah.

I liked Farrah's frosted, flipping hair that every haircutter in Queens called "wings" and her iconic orange swimsuit that accentuated her perkiness. She had a California tan that looked sunny and warm against my cool blue walls. By the end of every summer, after all those days at the swim club topped off by a week down in Florida, the sun-kissed glow I hoped to achieve resembled more of a baby-oiled, brown, peeling crisp. My gapless thighs still rubbed together, which was especially uncomfortable in the summer heat. The only thing Farrah and I had in common was that we shared a bedroom.

I was still a NARP (nonathletic, regular person) but looking less HercuLisa-like these days. Getting taller, thinning out, but still a bit fuller in the booty and thigh sections. There was a boy I crushed on in tenth grade and we eventually started dating. There was a popular song at the time, "Buffalo Gals," which he insisted on singing to me over and over again as he changed the lyrics to "Buffalo Butt." Yeah, it was meant to be funny, but I was not laughing inside. It was Patty all over again but this time more personal because I understood the depth of the insult in ways that I couldn't analyze when I was seven. Plus, he was supposed to care about me. We were dating!

This time, the comment fueled me as much as it hurt me. It was my "sand kicked in the face" moment. The old magic markers and sketch pads of days past would not provide an outlet for my unfavorable feelings like they used to. I was way too mad to draw. I took the bus home from one of our dates and got off a few stops early to walk home. I could feel my body walking faster and faster, feeding off all the feelings that were bottled up inside of me. My breath quickened. I walked and then I marched until sweat began to soak my shirt. Until my legs tingled from blood flow. Until I finally knocked enough sense back into me to decide that I was going to tell this boy to get lost.

One day, while cleaning the apartment, I found the dusty scale under Dad's dresser. Weighing yourself seemed to be what everyone was doing at the time, so I hopped on board. The number meant nothing; all I knew was that whatever it was, I was supposed to want it to be less. I'd weigh myself every morning to check in, waiting to see if the number had changed from 24 hours prior. I was never a numbers person and suddenly I was fixated on them. The size of my pants started to matter. I was concerned that the numbers on the leather patch of my Levi's would expose an unfavorable position, so my shirts were rarely tucked in. As I watched my dad continue to balloon to an even larger version of himself, the notion of ever being "fat" was taking on bigger meaning. Three simple letters with so much potential impact for a young girl.

I was beginning to see how much personal power I had to do the absolute opposite of my father. I was becoming more conscious of my body, my food choices, and my actions. It made me feel extremely powerful to have a say about what I was eating. I began to discover things we never kept in our fridge—yogurt with fruit, salads made with dark lettuce. I remember going to a friend's beach house for the weekend and her mom served us enormous cantaloupes cut in half with heaping scoops of cottage cheese inside the caverns. And that was all we ate until dinner. My stomach ached the entire afternoon in a way I wasn't used to. As we jumped the ocean waves and doused ourselves in baby oil, I felt the pang of hunger. I was too shy to ask about lunch, and if my friend and her mom weren't eating, then how could I complain? Her mom drank coffee all day, dropping pellets of sugar-free chemicals into the black liquid to sweeten it, she said, "without the calories." *Calories.* That was another new word for me. Food didn't control people at the Hamptons; they were in charge.

I went back to Flushing from my posh weekend feeling like I had been let in on the secret to a Hollywood lifestyle. Endless coffee, not much food, lots of sun. Back at home, I became even more disgusted by the boxed cakes and cookies piled on the kitchen table, and the hot dogs crackling on the indoor portable grill. For the first time, I felt revolted by many of the foods I had grown up on. TV dinners in foil trays that went straight from freezer to oven to snack table, canned stringed beans limp from sitting in water since the last world war, and bags of cookies that left your fingertips slippery from saturated fat. Yet, you'd think we owned a bunny because, despite the processed food, there were always carrots and a head of iceburg lettuce in the fridge. I munched on those instead, but I was so darn hungry. I didn't understand how the Hamptons could keep this up. I liked food way too much for this routine to sustain itself. Eventually, I volunteered to do the food shopping every week; if I could walk the aisles at the market, then I could pick out some things that were healthier.

Simultaneously, I began to experiment more with my dumbbell gift. The most innate thing to do was to pick them up and start curling like I had seen Dad do countless times. I curled and curled until, suddenly, I could feel something going on under my skin. It felt warm, crawly, tight. At first it felt odd, like a blood pressure cuff strangling my arm. The pulsing sensation under my skin made me feel weird. My imagination would run amok as I pictured bloody scenes in bad made-for-television movies. I recounted the day when my mother took me to the hospital to get stitches on my finger that I cut deeply in a high school sculpting class and she fainted at the sight of my blood. The doctors whisked her into the emergency room before me.

As I kept curling, the pulse of my own blood pumping in my veins became more pronounced. But then I felt how this tightness would quickly settle down after each set. I had never paid this much attention to how my body felt because of a simple, purposeful action. I could set my own body aflame with just weights and movement, and then witness the fire cooling down, all in a matter of seconds. It was the ultimate power.

When I was a kid, if your muscles hurt, you had a charley horse. But now this was no muscle cramp—this was intentional discomfort caused by tearing up my muscles, which is exactly what weight training does. The repetition of weights works the muscles and muscle fibers, making microscopic tears and then, when the tears heal back together, the muscle grows bigger and stronger. This resulted in muscle soreness the day after exercising. What a new sensation! It wasn't pain, like in having something fall on your head. This pain from exercise validated that I worked my body hard. I could power me.

After a few months of curling those weights, I began to notice my arms looking different. Petite peaks were forming on the part that Dad had labeled "biceps" in his little black book. I'd flex my arm and run my hand over the little bump thinking, *I made this*. It was odd to think that there was something underneath my skin that was waiting to surface. All I had to do was activate it. Up until this age in my life, I had grown in height, simply because my body was set to do so. With exercise, I was discovering the direct impact I had on my body because of my actions.

More and more, I was asking Dad for workout tips and leafing through his exercise magazines and personal notes for ideas. I even felt like maybe he was getting back into exercise, too, for a little while. He would demonstrate the movements, showing me lunges to work my legs, overhead presses to shape my shoulders, and French curls to set the backs of my arms on fire. I quickly learned how to maximize those little dumbbells to work my entire body. Eugen Sandow was right about how versatile a pair of dumbbells could be. There wasn't much room to do these movements in the bedroom I shared with my sister, so I opted for the living room in front of the TV, which I barely watched anymore except for a quality documentary such as *Pumping Iron*.

Pumping Iron was about the world of professional bodybuilding, which was gaining mainstream popularity at the time. It followed the rivalry between two main competitors, Lou Ferrigno (who, years later, became TV's "The Hulk") and Arnold Schwarzenegger (who, decades later, became the governor of California!), as they prepare for the 1975 IFBB Mr. Olympia competition in Pretoria, South Africa. Arnold stole the spotlight with his over-the-top personality, huge confidence and unbelievable physique. With a heavy Austrian accent, he'd talk about "the pump" and the feeling of blood rushing into your veins when you work out. This "pump" that Arnold was referring to was what I had been experiencing when working with my new dumbbells. Now, I understood it had a name!

I was learning how overhead shoulder presses could add natural contour to my frame. (A welcome option for achieving the look that huge shoulder pads of the time created.) Squats and lunges while holding dumbbells shaped my legs and bootie. I was becoming bilingual, quickly picking up a language that included words such as sets, reps (repetitions), tris (triceps), bis (biceps), lats (latissimus dorsi), pecs (pectoralis major), delts (deltoids), traps (trapezius), quads (quadriceps), hammies (hamstrings), ripped, pumped, and knurling (the gritty part of a barbell that gives it traction, making it easier to grip). There was something about the feeling of working my muscles, the tightness of "the pump," and the witnessing of physical change over time, that I loved.

This art of dabbling quickly morphed into a focus. I found it all so interesting, and stimulating, both physically and mentally. Plus, it gave Dad and I a unique shared interest to talk about together. I could feel our bond strengthening through a love of iron.

I was 16 years old, realizing that I could impact this thing that, up until then, I was quick to ridicule: my body. The fitness cork had been popped. I had spent the last few years gathering the carbonated bubbles—the hurtful words, the confusion, the lack of control, the tummy knots, the pondering of what it meant to be HercuLisa—to finally feel the pop. While learning how to work out my body, I was discovering how to connect with it, manipulate it, ignore it, and even like it.

Seeing that my interest in fitness was taking off, Dad got me a few exercise tapes to play on our newfangled VCR. I moved the snack tables aside to give myself space in the living room to do leg lifts and grapevines. Women in striped leggings, pink leotards, and sweatbands around fluffy '80s hair led me through exercise movements I had never seen before. Plus, it was all set to music. This was fun! It was my first taste of a structured workout class. A precise time frame where I actually—on purpose—did things to work my muscles, raise my heart rate, and break a sweat.

As a child, my food choices were a Whopper from Burger King or a Big Mac from McDonald's. Now my eyes were scanning different sections at the market: the dairy aisle where there were more choices than the transparent, bluish skim milk I was raised on. I was discovering cottage cheese, cottage cheese with pineapple, and nonfat yogurts. The cookie and cracker aisle had choices labeled "fat-free," which was trending. The fat-free items tasted like chemicals, but because lower calories were everyone's goal, my taste buds learned to adapt.

The longer I paid attention to what I was eating, and the more I curled those golden dumbbells and grapevined through my living room, the more I felt the cultivation of my power. Hearing Patty's voice as she counted my tummy rolls was feeding an inner beast I didn't even know existed.

One spring day, I suddenly had the urge to leave the apartment and run. Kids were always running away on TV, tying their things up in a cloth that they attached to a long stick flung over a shoulder. *Where were they going? Where was I going?* I had no way of articulating at the time that it was probably away from the walls of my small apartment that felt like they were closing in on me the older I got. The bedroom I shared with my sister was stiflingly small for two people. Our one and only bathroom was always occupied by someone other than me. There was hardly a place to go for a little privacy. My cat had the right idea by hiding under the bed most of the time. So, instead, I ran down Kissena Boulevard. I ran on the sidewalk, dodging people and the city-living chaos. I didn't consider running in the street, with all the buses and irritated drivers whizzing by. At first, I ran as far as the Brooklyn Conservatory. One block. Next time, I made it to Skyline Swim Club. Four blocks. Then to the Y, eight blocks, until finally I had made it as far as Kissena Park, the place where my grandmother would drive us to on the weekends because it was too far to walk. It felt like it was a world away. But it was only a mile, and I had just run it!

The mile was a guesstimate because I did not have a wearable or app to track it. Instead, I went by the "or so" theory. Twenty city blocks or so typically equaled a mile. It may have taken 15-20 minutes because, back then, my run pace was more of a shuffle-in-your-slippers pace, but it was more effort than just casual walking. I traversed the busy streets to the quieter, tree-lined sections near the park. Victorious in knowing that I just ran, nonstop, for 25 minutes. *You did it!* Unfortunately, I totally forgot about the turning around and going home part. I didn't run back the first time; I walked, slowly and calmly, as I thought about what I wanted to eat when I got home. Something crunchy like carrots, not chips. Something fresh, not canned.

I felt great when I was exercising. I loved the rush of adrenaline and how it propelled me in ways I had never seen myself before. I loved a good, hard-earned sweat. I loved the aftermath of sore muscles the next day. I loved pushing myself. I loved the connection between what I did and what I ate and how it resulted in my morphing physique. My tummy was flattening, my arms shaping, and my booty taking on a rounder, firmer form. The transformation was accelerated by the good food I was consuming. The more I exercised, the more I craved healthy foods. I was establishing a positive cycle between exercise and diet. Plus, I was having fun! It was a time in my life when everything felt moderately out of control, and to take charge of me through physical activity was empowering.

It was when I got my first job at the local Y that my life really started *working out*. The Y was about a half mile from my house, yet I never noticed it before. When stepping out onto Kissena Blvd from my building, all destinations pointed right: school, the subway, department stores, supermarkets, McDonald's, Dad's dental office. There was no need to go left except for dance class, the Skyline Swim Club, or Kissena Park. Now that I was running in that direction, I was passing the King Kullen food store, Chinese take-out, Lorabie's old-fashioned bakery where they tied strings around the cake boxes, apartment buildings that looked like mine, attached homes with tiny green lawns and small picket fences. I had passed the Y over and over again, watching people going in and out in exercise clothes, until, one day, out of curiosity, I went inside. Running through the streets of Flushing alone, with no music in my ears because nothing techy existed yet, I was discovering the world outside to the left of my door. I was discovering me. There was so much noise, yet I felt a newfound sense of quiet inside.

I got my first real-paying job at the Y helping out as a counselor at the after-school programs and summer camps. Granted, I made about two cents per hour, but I didn't care. I was proud of the paychecks made out to my name that I had to bring to the bank to deposit into my account. *My account.* I felt so grown up. After a few months of working at the Y, I was given an opportunity to start teaching an after-school class called the Junior Janies. I coined the name and designed the class. It was basically a babysitting job, but I was allowed to add my creativity to it, so I turned it into a fitness class for kids. I replicated some of the original aerobic videotape moves I had learned into a 30-minute class for kids five-to-seven years old. We did grapevines and leg lifts and lots of jumping to keep the sillies going while we exercised.

The Y had a well-equipped weight room, a huge gymnasium filled with the sounds of screeching sneakers, and the overall smell of sweat and chlorine. There was an indoor pool, which gave me a whole other perspective on swimming. Unlike Skyline, which was all about sun and fun and cannonballs and splashing (which technically wasn't allowed, so the lifeguards would dock us for a few minutes if we did), the people in this pool were rhythmic, lap-driven, and focused on their strokes.

The weight room was not much bigger than my parents' bedroom where my dad tinkered with his weights. There were mirrors on the walls, some cracked and taped together. Benches with greasy-looking plastic upholstery and jagged tears on the cushions that exposed yellowed stuffing. A few archaic-type machines that looked like apparatus for torturing the enemy. Contraptions with funky handles and oddly placed padding. And included in most of these machines were flat, rectangular weights stacked one on top of the other with numbers on them—40, 50, 60…180, 200—and a metal pin to select your choice. These numbers equaled pounds.

And then there were free weights, just like Dad's. Countless pairs of corroded dumbbells, some black, some gray, all with a rusty amber dusting that eventually worked its way onto my T-shirts and sweats like fast-lane skid marks. The dumbbell sizes ranged from the ones that Dad got me all the way up to those as big as a Volkswagen. The dainty, light weights (five pounds, like my gold ones) collected dust in the corner as I observed that most of the people coming in and out of the weight room were men.

By now I was 17 years old, and this environment should have intimidated a soft-spoken, slightly introverted, artsy-fartsy person like me. But I secretly liked being one of the only girls in the room. It made me feel quite HercuLisa-esque. No one seemed to be judging me or anyone else for that matter. Every person was focused on individual efforts. Even if I was just using the five-pound weights, hanging out with the guys made me feel good about myself. They talked differently than girls. Said what they meant. Didn't turn their backs to huddle and whisper.

I was picking up on all the quirky gym nuances, from the smorgasbord of equipment to the eclectic mix of members. Gyms are notorious for attracting a funny crowd, and the members often get nicknames from the other members. There was Happy Howie, who was always clad in spandex shorts a size too small, a spandex top, and a red, white, and blue headband. Howie was always bopping from one machine to the next, doing jumping jacks in between, and curling dumbbells at a rapid pace. Panting like a dog. Sweat pouring from every orifice and, because his terry cloth headband was only able to catch the sweat from his brow, the rest of the downpour was left all over the machines. Sit Up Guy was the guy who did sit ups. Only sit ups. Like thousands of them in a row. He also ran in a circle, not the track—but a circle the size of a hula hoop—in the gymnasium for a half hour straight.

And there was this cute guy with a baseball cap who was always at the Y. I assumed he worked there. He was always walking the halls, going into offices, talking to everyone, and constantly eating out of plastic deli containers. Macaroni salad or coleslaw. Some kind of white, creamy stuff you'd bring to a barbeque. We made eye contact one day. He smiled; I smiled. I asked someone his name. I went home and told my sister all about the cute guy at the Y whose last name sounded something like "saccharine."

One spring day, the cute guy and I talked for hours on the front steps of the Y. He was 19 years old, organized all the basketball leagues, and worked at summer sports camp. He lived in the apartment building across the street. Mr. Super Jock. Basketball player. Baseball player. A college boy. He talked about so many parts of his life, from his mother being bedridden for the last few years because of multiple sclerosis, to his two older brothers and his dad. He liked rock music. Italian food. Macaroni salad. Jokes. Drives.

We started working out together in the weight room every once in a while. He knew exercise terminology that I had never heard of before, such as physiology, kinesiology, and biomechanics. "Ologies" were not my thing. He understood how muscles worked, and which exercises were designed to work specific body parts. *Dad would love him!* I thought very early on. Our workouts together became more frequent. He was becoming the only person who knew when to push me to work a little harder in the gym. I knew how much to spot him on a bench press. When you spot someone, particularly on bench press, there's a fine line between helping too much (which means the lifter doesn't get the max benefit from the effort), and not helping enough (which can result in the lifter getting pummeled by the weight). It takes a while to figure out that space.

I had found my workout partner. The person who made me want to show up all the time and give it my all. The one who relied on me as much as I counted on him. The guy who treated me like the most important person in the world. Plus, he never once told me I had a "buffalo" gluteus maximus.

Craig.

Craig was the most competitive person I had ever met. Everything he attempted, athletically, came to him with little effort. Basketball, tennis, volleyball, shuffleboard—if there was a round, movable object involved, Craig was king of the court. I, on the other hand, threw a ball like my arm was an overcooked noodle. My eyes could be focused straight ahead on my target, yet the ball always landed in a bush. I envied the girls who could whip a softball to their boyfriends or flip a Frisbee so hard it could take the paint off a car.

We were the stereotypical "High School Musical" couple (except we were now in college—both at Queens College—me a freshman, him a junior). He was the jock who couldn't carry a tune, even if it had a handle. Even though I was getting into exercise, I was still the artsy one, gravitating toward things like writing, drawing, and singing. Craig could run seven-minute miles, shoot three-point shots, dribble a ball between his legs, spike a ball, kick a ball, throw a ball—with power, precision, and speed. The only thing I had over him in a physical sense, aside from my foundation in dance, which did offer a tad of gracefulness, was swimming. Somehow, despite being exposed to every sport imaginable, Craig never learned to swim. While I was splashing around all summer at Skyline, Craig was crouched down in catcher position, sweating in a polyester uniform, on a baseball field under the burning sun. Finally, I could beat him at something! But showing off your sidestroke, which is probably the least impressive stroke yet was the one I did best, was not as easy as picking up a ball and hurling it across a field.

Neither of us learned to ride bikes, which made us even there. I had a bike when I was really little. Banana seat, plastic wicker basket, training wheels—the works. When it was time to take the trainers off, my nervous mom, who had heard that some neighborhood girl broke her leg when she hit a sidewalk crack while riding her bike, took my entire bike away instead.

Any sport Craig tossed my way, I was willing to try even though it usually ended with me in tears. We could have been goofing around on the basketball court, shooting foul shots, and he was still egging me on. Every ball I shot and missed, he scored and made sure I knew it. *Nah-nah-nah-nah-nah.* When I lifted a weight, he had to double it. He took me to the track for the first time in my life, and when I could barely run around once at his pace, I was completely humbled. And mad. He was scrappy. I was skipping. He was cut-throat. I was butter knife. He loved to tease me about my lack of athleticism. That would make me mad and I'd try a little harder. But the perseverance only lasted so long. Eventually, frustration led to defeat…and more tears.

All those casual jogs to the park, and all those hours of aerobic workouts in my living room, were pivotal steps toward making fitness a part of my regular routine. Still, I had no idea I had only grazed the surface. Unlike teens today who are involved in sports and exercise since they were practically in diapers, I had no "formal training" in anything athletic. Craig, however, helped me raise my fitness bar to an entirely new level. His teasing and competitiveness may have made me want to kill him at times, but it was the push toward my personal brink that brought out something in me that I had never seen before. I wasn't used to pushing. Feeling physically uncomfortable on purpose was not familiar to me. Like that burning stitch you get in your side from running as fast as you can. Or the feeling of your heart thumping so hard you think it could pop out of your chest. Nor did I understand the feeling of arriving victoriously on the other side of the push. Victory was all about position of place.

Between Craig's teasing and cajoling, I discovered my personal gas tank. I hadn't been reading my fuel gauge at all. I didn't even know it existed. Plus, I was discovering that, when I felt mad or frustrated, I could dip even deeper into a power inside of me and make my body do something with it. While journaling helped me sort through the feelings, it never made me feel physically strong. Exercise helped me convert the frustration, anger, disappointment, and confusion—basically, life—into personal power.

It was a few years since we first talked on the steps at the Y, and Craig and I were a bona fide couple. Very much into each other and connected at the hip through our day-to-day lives, which included going to school, work, and working out. Our first year as a couple seemed to roll by. Whether it was shooting baskets at the park, training in the weight room at school, slapping a handball against the side of my apartment building, or walking the two miles home from campus instead of taking the bus, we did something active together almost every single day. It was through exercise that we really got to know each other. While we were always on different fitness levels, our relationship was built on a partnership in exercise. You learn a lot about people when you train with them. Craig and I were quickly figuring out that we were good together—in and out of the gym.

In college, I double majored in communications and English; Craig majored in physical education. Most of my classes were on one end of the campus in buildings with camera equipment, theater stages, and geeky English professors who really did wear tweed blazers with suede elbow patches. Craig's classes were on the other end, in and around the Fitz gymnasium where rubber soles squeaked against shiny linoleum floors and the air reeked of sweat and chlorine. Having a serious boyfriend who was always at the gym (for class or team practice) meant I spent a lot of time there, too. If I thought the Y was an incredible place to exercise, my perception of "amazing" was redefined with the gym at college. Instead of two machines for legs, there were eight. There wasn't just one row of dumbbells to choose from; there were six. I hopped onto machines I had never heard of—Smith machine, abductor/adductor machine, hack press. It was exercise heaven.

Hanging around with college athletes gave me a taste of what it meant to exercise with intensity and purpose. These people weren't just looking for "the pump"; sports were a major part of their college experience. Craig played on the basketball and baseball teams, so I met tons of athletes. I was impressed by the things they could do with their bodies—how fast they could run, how high they could jump, and how much they could persevere.

Everyone was always clicking stopwatches, measuring distances, and high-fiving each other. They wore team uniforms and jackets with names and nicknames embroidered over their hearts. They practiced their sport for hours after school and then went out to dinner together, only to get up the next morning for an early workout or a stretching session with the athletic trainer. I had never seen a community of such intense people bonded by a common goal that hinged on what their bodies could do. And their bodies all looked so amazing! Muscular and toned, washboard abs, bulging calves. Even their hands and forearms were in shape evidenced by muscle striations that surfaced with the simplest moves, like picking up a backpack. And when they were working out or competing in their sport, they all had this look in their eyes. A focus, a stare, an intensity— like they were looking at something I couldn't see. I knew about the "Eye of the Tiger" from the movie *Rocky*; I had just never seen it up close and in person.

I was exposed to seeing just how much the body could do if the mind was willing to fight for it. Seeing these athletes challenge themselves, when it appeared there wasn't a drop left in the tank, simply amazed me. They huffed and puffed like mad dogs. Sweat poured off their faces. Their facial expressions captured pain and determination. I wanted to be a part of all *this* and I wasn't even sure I understood what it was. These people had swagger, attitude, drive, muscles. I didn't just want to be Craig's artsy English major girlfriend. I wanted to be a part of this elite warrior pack.

In the spring of my freshman year, I tried out for the women's track team. I liked to run. I liked being outside. The weather was beautiful. *What the heck?*

First day out, I stood on the track with a group of female athletes. These women were beasts—beautiful, tall, lean, muscular runners who were wearing spandex shorts and fitted tank tops. They reeked of intensity. Of people who eat people like me for breakfast. The coach gave an inspirational welcome-to-the-team talk. Everyone stood around with their hands perched toughly on their waists the way athletes do. I stressed over where exactly to place my hands: *Do I go with the exact small of my waist? Or lower down around the hips?*

Coach clapped his hands really loud and shouted, "Now let's get out there and warm up! Four times around and we'll meet back here to stretch out." A whistle blew. Something in my brain snapped and then my thoughts began to race even before my legs: *Did he just say four times? That's a mile! That's half of the biggest run I've ever done in my life!* I felt panic take over as everyone bolted. Pride kept my feet going; fear kept my mind racing. *What the heck did I sign up for?*

That night, I put ice packs on my burning shins and thought about the next workout just 24 hours away. After one week of daily two-hour practices, I felt shot beyond any physical fatigue I had ever experienced. My body ached to the core. My feet hurt. My abs hurt. My big toenail was black. Every night, I'd crawl into bed, only to wake up to the reality that I had practice again that afternoon. My pride was equally bruised. I wasn't fast. I didn't have endurance. I was so out of my element.

As I ran each afternoon, usually alone because most of my teammates were way ahead, I felt my mind doing laps around my inner dialogue. *You can't do this. You suck at this. You're always in last place. Why are you doing this? What are you trying to prove?* The more I entertained doubt, the more I could feel my pace slowing down. After two weeks of running more mileage than I ever had, and experiencing the worst physical pain of my life, I quit the team. I convinced myself that, with school work and a part-time job at a real estate office, I didn't have time for a team sport. Truth was, I was tired of feeling bad about me.

Craig was understanding. He pointed out that many of the other women had been running since they were little kids. He reminded me that they were built for running with long legs, lean muscle mass, and lots of fast-twitch fibers. He didn't make me feel bad for quitting track. "You should lift more," he said. "You're naturally strong."

I had quit track.

I had quit ballet.

I had quit me.

Quitters are not strong.

Maybe I did have tenacity, but it was short-lived. The spark of drive that I had felt when faced with a challenge or a ribbing from Craig only lasted while at the precipice of my emotion.

Anyone can get mad at something or about something, and growl back at it. The strength and drive come from the extended push. I didn't know how to do that part yet. Being able to persevere through the hard parts—those moments when the adrenaline rush has subsided—is when the actual work happens.

But Craig was right; I did like to lift, and I was decently strong *for a girl*. Weight training required very little skill. Just pick it up, put it down. Press it up, control it down. Pull it down, control it up. Simple. No points to accumulate. No teammates to disappoint. No places to come in (like last). When you weight train, if you can push all the noise aside, it's just about you and the iron. I could crawl inside myself, lift the dumbbells, and not worry if I was doing it wrong or letting someone down. I saw that I could push past a bad feeling, like a burning sensation inside a muscle, and get just one more rep. I was beginning to create a personal paradigm shift.

Mental drive was not enough. Just wanting something was the spark, but it was the mental *control* that began to take me from point A to point B. I was slowly increasing my weights, like picking up the 15-pound dumbbells instead of the 10-pound ones. I could test myself over and over again, going for 12 repetitions instead of 10, without anyone ever knowing about these mini tests. Having it all unfold inside my own thoughts made me feel like I was building an invisible fortress. No one knew if I failed or succeeded. I was training my mind just as hard as my body. The more I trained with weights, the more compelled I was to train with weights. Weeks turned into months; months turned into a year. After a year of serious weight training, at a schedule of four to five times per week for an hour each time, I felt different. I looked different. My body weight was heavier than ever, and I loved that because I knew muscle weighs more than fat.

For me and Craig, lifting was also entertainment, like going to a movie or shopping at the mall. We loved lifting, and we especially loved doing it together. He'd do a set, I'd spot him. I'd do a set, he'd spot me. We developed an unspoken understanding of each other, from how much help the other needed to complete a repetition to exactly when to cheer the other one on or remain quiet. And even when Craig was acting all competitive in the gym, like who could do more reps on the last set, I could take it because I had finally found a fitness arena where I could keep up.

Eventually, we moved beyond the gyms at the Y and school and joined a regular gym, one where you had to pay for membership. No longer did we want to tack working out onto activities we were already engaged in, like work or academics. Going to a separate gym meant this was the beginning of a serious, more hardcore commitment to fitness. We were suddenly members of something—members of more than a place, but part of a community that would shape our bodies, our beliefs, and our friendships.

The first gym membership was to Diamond's Gym in College Point, New York. If I thought my college gym experience opened my eyes to fitness, Diamond's made my head explode.

Diamond's was in a huge warehouse, surrounded by other industrial buildings including a bakery, which seemed like a cruel joke because it always smelled like fresh-baked bread when we drove down the street. No matter how early in the morning or late in the evening, there were always members inside the gym. Parked cars lined the city street off the main drag, College Point Boulevard. Most cars were dilapidated, rusted clunkers, like ours. A rare few were sleek red convertibles with vanity license plates like MRHUGE. These were the ones that always managed to find a spot right in front of the building. The lofted ceilings were met with casement windows covered in dirt where people would write in the grime things like "Lift or Die." The peel-and-stick letters on the front glass door had more peel than stick. The powerful smells of body odor, Ben Gay, and a musty, woodsy, protein-powdered health food store scent lingered each day in the stale air. Monday nights were the busiest of days at the gym when people would redeem themselves from a weekend of partying at the dance clubs on Bell Boulevard or cruising Francis Lewis Boulevard in their cars until the sun rose.

It was my first exposure to hardcore lifting. There were guys with bulging, rippled pecs bursting out of skin so filo-dough thin that you could see cross-striations in the muscles and veins expanding with blood with each repetition. "The pump" in action! The women looked nothing like the prissy ladies clad in leggings and leg warmers in my exercise tapes. These women, and there were only a few of them in the gym, were just as no-frills and hardcore as the men. They wore clingy tank tops and frayed sweatshirts with necklines cut low enough to hang off one shoulder. No cute pops of color headbands or fanciful socks draped over high-top aerobic sneakers.

With heavy lifting came heavy metal and hard rock music. AC/DC, Poison, Metallica, and Queen played on a continuous loop on the highest volume possible. "Thunderstruck" was our theme song for squats. "Back in Black" epitomized deadlifts. "Welcome to the Jungle" was perfect for warming up. These songs became our lifting anthems and, in true Pavlovian style, hearing them—even while just driving to work—made my heart race. Weights clanking while loading plates and bars dropping to the ground with a last rep were the additional sound tracks to our favorite songs. No one wore headsets to pipe in personal tunes, so the entire gym worked out to one beat. This synergized the community, strengthening a cult-like atmosphere where all the members rocked out to the same song, in the same location, with the same goal: to get bigger and stronger.

There was music and, of course, mirrors. Mirrors covered every wall, so you could catch an angle of yourself at just about any point. Bodybuilders would lift their shirts in between sets to examine rippled abs, even if the set just completed was for arms. The mirrors were usually cracked from someone flinging a weight, and then taped together with silver duct tape because replacing them was not in the budget. I'm not really sure what *was* in the budget—stuff was old and run-down, rusted and grimy, and we loved it that way.

And layered on top of all the music and reflecting was the constant yelling: *Come on, push! One more! You got this! Do it!* Yelling at each other, yelling at yourself. Before closing time each night (Craig and I were usually there until the last second), the entire gym looked like a warzone. Weights scattered all over the floor, sweat streaks on every bench and cushion, forgotten sweatshirts piled in corners, and the overall stench of hard work. These were the signs of a good day in our world of working out.

We had been pouring through books and magazines to design our workouts. Legs one day, arms another, chest and back, shoulders, heavy days, rep days. We were discovering different ways to work a muscle from the center or the sides, me never realizing before that a muscle group could have that many entry points. There were methods behind each workout, like the yin-yang of a "push/pull" day (pushing for chest, pulling for back), or a "rep" (repetitions) day where we'd drop the pounds of the weights but increase the number of repetitions. We learned by watching veteran lifters, too, and by trial and error. The error part typically equaled a tweaked muscle or blood blister from catching a finger between a weight and a bar. Craig's Phys Ed background, rich in kinesiology and physiology, guided our efforts toward a more scientific approach for what we were doing to our bodies.

We also began to establish our workout crowd. Granted, most everyone was male, but because I was developing a reputation for training *like one of the guys*, it didn't bother them or me. Everyone had a regular name—Anthony, Drew, Pete, Sal, Steve, Mark. And then everyone had a nickname—Sweater Man (because he trained in a cardigan sweater with no shirt underneath), Dirty Harry (because he always wore the same dingy-gray, formerly white sweatpants), and The Bull (because he was built like one and was constantly screaming with his Russian accent "strong like bull!"). Craig was The Crane because he could deadlift ridiculous amounts.

Somehow, I got the nickname Tank. (I still hadn't shared the old HercuLisa name yet with anyone but Craig.) I had a reputation for being all business in the gym, lifting as heavy as I could, never complaining when something hurt, or if I felt like I was about to toss my cookies from pushing so hard. The workouts, and the entire gym comradery, gave me confidence in my body's ability to accomplish goals that I had never considered before. Like the way certain people can walk on their hands or do a backflip or dribble a ball. I was never one of those people. All my hands could do was create art. Now, I was learning even more how to push my body, move it, trust it, and ignore it. I was shedding my "nonathlete" persona. There was no weight that I wasn't willing to try to lift. I was beginning to believe in my body when for so long I was merely renting space inside of her. I was developing a confidence in myself at Diamond's Gym—an apropos name for a place where diamonds in the rough go to chisel their bodies into something of worth.

At Diamond's, we perfected basic lifts that netted tremendous gains in both strength and confidence. For example, squats. There's nothing like approaching a barbell loaded up with the biggest amount of weight you've ever attempted, staring it down, ducking under it, locking it into place on your back, popping it off the rack, stepping back with it while your chalked hands grip the coarse knurling for dear life, taking the biggest inhale you can muster, and holding that air until you feel like you might burst, looking up toward the sky in prayer that you are bigger than this weight, dropping down into the squat, getting down low enough to count as "contest depth" (top of your hip below the top of your knee; aka "ass to the grass"), and getting back up again only to drop it down again if you have the guts.

Do you have the guts?

Do you?

Do I?

YES, I DO!

All that dialogue taking place inside my head during the split second while breaking the bar from the rack because, once the actual squats begin, your brain goes to black. *Back in Black.* You hear nothing but the spotter screaming behind you. You see nothing, even though there's typically a cracked mirror right in front of you. You feel everything, from the crushing pain of having 225 pounds pressing across the top your back and traps, to the pressure inside your head because you're still holding your breath. Squats beat the crap of out lifters.

In addition to squats, the other basics were bench pressing and deadlifting. These three exercises were the components of a specific kind of sport called powerlifting. Our gym posse spent a lot of time powerlifting. One by one, we'd all rotate through a workout, sometimes four or five of us at a time, loading and unloading each other's weights and cheering each other on. While we were all very serious about the workouts, we also laughed a lot. We were establishing tons of inside jokes and building strong friendships with exercise at the core.

I was learning about exercise goals. About setting them, crushing them, and then raising the bar a little higher to reach another level of accomplishment. We were also becoming even more driven and focused, or, one might argue, obsessed. Craig had a part-time job as a fitness trainer at the BQE (which stood for the Brooklyn-Queens Expressway). It was a full-service, upscale fitness club that featured everything from an enormous weight room to racquetball courts to the fanciest locker rooms where you could help yourself to crisp white towels for the shower. If Craig worked the evening shift, I would meet him there at 11:30 pm so we could start working out when he was done at midnight. By the time we finished blasting a body part, it was close to 2 am.

One day, after a few months of doing powerlifting exercises and lots of research on what the competitive landscape looked like at the time, Craig said, "We should both compete in a powerlifting meet. Your lifts would totally blow away the competition."

Me? Compete? Blow away? None of that sounded like the Lisa I had known most of my life. But Tank, secretly aka HercuLisa? We were intrigued.

THE EARLY COMPETITIVE YEARS

Up until now, the grammar school Halloween art contest had been my one and only foray into competition. It was based on a natural talent that I didn't think much about or invest much energy into perfecting. I just liked to draw. My tools were pencils and paper. My inspiration came straight from my imagination. The stakes were pretty low and that worked great for me.

Competing in powerlifting intrigued me. It also terrified me. Sure, I lifted weights with intensity and power, but that didn't mean that I was a *powerlifter*. Like if you asked me, do I run? Yes. Am I a runner? Heck no. The "er" at the end of these words meant that I was accomplished. That I had earned the right to give myself a title. *What if you're not good enough to compete as a powerlifter? What if you can't?* The little voice in my head casted doubt, but the antithesis quickly chimed in to reverse the negativity: *What if you can?*

I mustered the courage to enter my first powerlifting meet. It was a few months away, giving me enough time to scout out another meet or two to see how it all worked, to practice lifting based on the judges' cues (like waiting for the signal to rack a weight instead of doing it at my own pace), to lift while donning special equipment such as a bench shirt or squat suit, and to try to get as strong as possible to be competitive.

While bench pressing is the mother of all chest exercises (it hits multiple parts of the pectorals, plus triceps), squatting is the king of leg exercises (quadriceps and hamstrings and even gluteus maximus). Deadlifts mostly work the back, legs and traps. Depending on whether you deadlift sumo style (legs wide apart) or conventional (legs close together), you also build hip and grip strength. And because powerlifting is a sport that forces you to engage your entire body to complete the lifts, the core (abdominals and back) is constantly at work. Core is exactly that—the center and foundation of your being. Like a large oak tree, equally strong and solid no matter which angle of it you're looking at and built with a quality interior that keeps the tree standing tall. While many people at the gym were gung ho about separately developing six-pack abs and a muscular back, and they would design workouts specific to those parts, core work from powerlifting built those sections simultaneously. Put all three exercises together—squatting, benching, and deadlifting—in one workout on one day and you've got yourself competitive powerlifting. Competitive powerlifters perform these three exercises for three attempts each for a potential of nine lifts in one given meet. Very different from training in the gym where you normally train squats one day and deadlifts on another.

Attempts are like reps, and you want to make sure that each rep is strategically geared toward the following: (a) getting your opener (aka your first lift, which helps to ensure you don't bomb out, which means you're disqualified from that meet) and (b) lifting your maximum weight.

Sometimes you don't get credit for an attempt (the judges say your squats are not deep enough, or your deadlift was "hitched," which means you dragged it up your thighs). Sometimes it's because you didn't have the strength that day and either got crushed under a bench press (the spotters had to lift the weight off your chest because you surely couldn't). Other reasons can include being unable to budge the bar off the ground in your deadlift. (It's humbling to roll the bar across the platform instead of pulling it up.) Or you might squat down like it's nobody's business and you simply cannot get back up. Not even an inch. Spotters have to catch you and the bar on your back (you hope it's still on your back!) with all the weights on that bar so you don't wind up on the floor. Basically, you just don't have it that day. It's crushing to the ego and body, but it's also just part of the sport. This is why they're called *attempts*. Props to the lifters for trying. Bless the spotters for catching. At the end of the meet, if you've managed to not bomb out, your heaviest attempt in each exercise is added up for a total of how much weight you lifted that day. The competitor who lifts the most in his or her age and/or weight class wins. Second place, third place, fourth place, and so forth, follow suit.

When I first started powerlifting, very few of my non-gym friends understood what it was. I barely did! Powerlifting always required a lengthy explanation accompanied by some physical gestures to demonstrate the moves. Most people were familiar with weightlifting, especially with its exposure in the Olympics (aka Olympic lifting). I would explain: "No, weightlifting is different. That's a snatch, and clean and jerk. Powerlifting is a squat, bench press, and deadlift. You put a bar on your back, loaded with weight, and squat down deep for one repetition. No, not the lift that you throw up over your head. That's weightlifting." At this point, I would drop to the floor to mime the moves of a bench press. Flat on my back, I would pretend to lift a bar off my chest straight up in the air. I would explain that the bar needed to pause and steady itself on the chest (note: there are lots of rules to know when you lift in a powerlifting meet) until a judge yelled, "Press!"

For the deadlift demonstration, I would pop back up on my feet and bend down to lift an imaginary bar from the floor to a standing position. I would explain the importance of waiting for the proper cues from the judges, such as "down," because, if I didn't, the lift could be disqualified. And how it was the lifter's goal to lift as much weight as possible.

"How much can you lift?" It was always the question du jour. People are numbers oriented; they just want to know. During my competitive powerlifting years, my very best was a 330-pound squat, 185-pound bench press, and 365-pound deadlift (conventional style). My weight class fluctuated between 123 pounds and 139 pounds.

My first powerlifting meet was run by the ADFPA (American Drug-Free Powerlifting Association). Drug-free was a critical criterion for me and Craig. While I never saw lifters actually injecting drugs into their bodies, I knew steroid use was real. Doors would close at the gym for private meetings between staff and members. Steroid users were usually easy to spot. Insane strength, massive muscle size, random rage (like when an exercise machine had the "Out of Order" sign on it and they would throw a weight across the room), and angry-looking purple pimples all over their backs. There were a few women who were built like men and with baritone voices. Some people were overt about their steroid use, while others fell into the *don't ask, don't tell* mode. I didn't have a problem with their lifestyle choices; I just didn't want to compete against them.

If I participated in a nondrug-tested competition, it meant that I would most likely be up against women who were using performance enhancing drugs. And, therefore, I would get crushed! While my 365-pound deadlift was competitive in a drug-free meet, it could get blown away by nondrug-tested meets where women were deadlifting in the mid-400s! Drug use scared me. With drug-free competition came drug testing, so I had to get used to peeing in a cup in bathrooms at meet sites while an official stood watching.

From the moment of my first lift in this first competition, which started promptly at 10 am, to my last lift around 3 pm, my adrenaline was pumping. Each time the announcer called, "Lisa Safran, in the hole" (which means two lifters are in front of me to do their lifts, so I should be getting ready to go)…"Lisa Safran, on deck" (one lifter in front of me)…"Up next, Lisa Safran" (my turn!)…, my heart rate skyrocketed.

I donned all the lifting gear, including a super-tight squat suit, equally tight bench shirt, tourniquet-tight knee wraps, wrist wraps, and a sturdy, suede-covered weightlifting belt. The items were made of the thickest, stiffest, toughest materials, with heavy stitching in strategic places, and there was zero give to the fabric. On purpose! The tight gear held your body together like a cannon stuffed with ammunition, and the moment of explosion was the lift. For example, if you were squatting, the knee wraps offered spring action and support to help you stand back up with the weight. Designed to help athletes lift heavier loads, the gear was a necessary evil.

Getting these clothes on your body took a village. Imagine the fierce effort you need to release the bottom of a tucked in blanket when sleeping in a hotel bed. That's how hard it was to get the gear on. Craig would help me squeeze myself into lifting suits that left tender welts where the creases of the garment dug deeply into my hips and thighs. Tugging and yanking on the garment and pulling up the straps, actually lifting me off the floor at times like a marionette on a stage, until it was finally fully on. The worst was the bench shirt. When I put one on for the first time, the pain actually made me cry. The material dug deeply into my armpits when I performed the bench press movement, feeling like a rope ripping into my flesh. But as the team would say at the gym, *Don't be a Mary*, which translated to "don't act like a girl." So, for the greater gain of a heavier bench press, I was no *Mary*. The knee wraps went around my knees so many times and so tightly that I could barely walk to the platform without looking like Frankenstein. If your legs take on a tinge of blue from cutting off circulation, you know you're wrapped well.

Everything about a powerlifting competition, from the energy of the other competitors to the very private place in my mind where I would crawl into right before the lift, put my entire being on fire. The scent of Tiger Balm (it's like Ben Gay, only stronger) stoked the fire. A popped ammonia cap waved under my nose right before a lift made me feel like screaming. Weights clanking and lifters shouting created sounds I could latch onto. The feeling of lifting chalk in my sweaty, calloused palms meeting the cold metal bar was as exhilarating as diving head first into a pile of a season's first snowfall.

In this first meet, I squatted 225 pounds, benched 135 pounds, and deadlifted 310 pounds for a total of 670 pounds in the 129-pound women's division. These were the heaviest weights I had ever lifted. At the end of the meet, as the placements were announced, I heard my name along with the word *winner*. To my surprise, I took first place in my class. I was handed a gold 18-inch trophy with a woman holding a barbell at the top of her deadlift, standing on a sturdy black base with an engraved plaque. She was the female counterpart to the *David* statue. I was bursting with pride, confidence, and a sense of accomplishment. I couldn't wait to tell Dad.

This single competition flipped a switch in me. I literally felt so strong—from my muscles to my mind and to the invisible current that connected those two parts. My strength was totally mine, and yet strangely based on everyone else's: the other lifters, the judges, the spectators, the other members in the gym, Craig. My blinders were on, forcing me to focus only on the goal in front of me, yet I fed off the cheers of the crowd and the energy of my fellow competitors and teammates.

So, what do you do when you're a powerlifter who has been bitten by the competition bug? You enter more competitions, you train harder, you aim to push past what you thought was your previous best. Train, compete, repeat. You become the tube of toothpaste that you swear is fully squeezed out and done, but somehow you manage to roll out one more brushing.

I headed back to the gym with a vengeance, ready to invest more sweat equity toward my goals. The workouts were grueling, because with every competition completed came the desire to do better next time. And the only way to raise the competitive bar was to push harder, work longer, dig deeper, and test my physical and mental strength more than the time before. My body was willing to take on anything I would throw at it. The more I pushed it, the quicker I saw results. It became a wonderfully fulfilling cycle. The body that I spent so many years growing into, and often fighting against, was finally something I understood, respected, and relied on. I would just show up at the gym, day after day, get under a barbell, and lift.

Monday nights were squat workouts. I'd wake up every Monday with the same sick, excited feeling in my stomach that I was going to have to face the bar that night. Of all the lifts, squats hurt the most. Your back hurts, your legs burn, your shoulders cry out for mercy as they work to support the bar; and if you're cinching a stiff lifting belt around your core for maximum back support, you're dying from that. Squats, and I mean full, all-the-way-down-past-parallel squats, separate men from mice. A deep squat engages your muscles and makes your body work, plus it prepares you for competition when you're judged on your squat depth. It means you're not cheating yourself, like reading the Cliffs Notes instead of the original Shakespearean play.

Every week, the goal was to push a little harder than the week before with either more reps or more weight. The good thing about squatting on Mondays was that I had taken off Sunday and felt fully rested. The bad thing was that I was fully rested. Rest made my "Eye of the Tiger" less piercing. It gave my chronically sore body a chance to kick back. This was terrible for my psyche! I was beginning to tune into just how easy it was for my workouts to get sabotaged by my own head games.

Tuesdays were for chest and benching. I always looked forward to benching. It was the exercise where I saw my best gains, albeit slow and steady. The markers of my success were represented by which plates were on the bar. Even when I was adding a wafer-thin 2.5-pound plate on each side (these were the smallest *Mary* weights in the gym), I knew I was chipping away at a bigger goal. It took months of consistent training before I graduated to full-fledged 25-pound plates, and then a few years before I slapped on the big boys—45-pound plates. If you saw a woman benching with these monsters tacked onto each end of the bar, she had arrived as a lifter. "How much do you bench?" It was like little kids in the playground asking each other their age. The bigger the number, the better. Over the years, I progressed my 135-pound "PR" bench press (this is the weight of the bar and one big 45-pound plate on each side) to reps of 10. And my new "PR" in a meet became 185 pounds. ("PR" = personal record).

Wednesdays were reserved for shoulders, Thursdays for deadlifts, Fridays for arms, Saturdays for a hodgepodge of body parts to hit again, and Sundays for rest. Having a dedicated, regimented schedule kept me focused and on point.

Based on my workouts in the gym, I had an idea what poundage I was capable of in my next meet. If all went as planned, I could possibly do even a little more in the competition because of the adrenaline factor. But here's the thing: all rarely went as planned. My bench might have been rocketing, but my squat was off. My deadlift was on course for a "PR," but then I'd get tweaked a week before competition. The perfect recipe for the perfect meet was that all three lifts were simultaneously progressing, that I had remained injury-free, and that I was not getting my period the morning of the meet. (It's not fun to compete with cramps, plus the bloat can mess with making a weight class.) Training may be a science, something you can methodically map out, but the art of ever-changing life scenarios, like getting a bad head cold the night before competition, makes all the planning feel like a joke. The real grit comes from how well you power through the challenges.

All this training and competing was transforming my body. I was becoming thick in the middle from building a solid, muscular core, and whatever girlish taper I had was disappearing. My trapezius muscles popped out from all the deadlifts and my arms were meaty with muscle. Even my booty had morphed into a full, anything-but-small squatter's butt, which was a good thing. A source of power! Even more, I looked nothing like the girls in my old teen magazines, and, at this point, that thrilled me. I felt athletic. Invincible. Strong.

As my fitness connection continued to accelerate, and I was sharing more and more of my progress with Dad, I could see that he was less immersed in his own. My mom had been recently diagnosed with Parkinson's disease, making their day-to-day lives overwhelming at times. The last thing on his mind was his own exercise. The chest of weights was now a table top for newspapers and packages. His body weight seemed to be creeping up, evidenced by the need to start wearing suspenders because his belts weren't making it around his belly any more. While my sister and I did all we could to support our parents in their daily lives, I couldn't erase their struggle. And, at the time, I saw it as so physical. Dad was getting larger and slowing down. Mom was losing her ability to do simple tasks like button her own frilly blouse. Just getting through an average day seemed like all they could manage. Dad had given me the fitness torch for my sixteenth birthday, a torch he struggled so hard to keep ignited for himself. I was determined to stay physical for the two of us, for all of us.

I would tell Dad everything I was doing in the gym, describing all the newfangled equipment that he would have loved to try. He would eat it up. He'd squeeze my biceps when I flexed. I showed him my trophies. He would share exercise knowledge with my workout partner, who was already a fixture around our house, and I could see them developing a bond through iron. Dad was a wealth of fitness know-how from the old-school days when bodybuilding was just taking off. Craig had a strong science background from his recently acquired physical education degree. They were an intelligent duo. Mom's health continued to deteriorate, so staying connected to the exercise world via my experiences seemed to be a healthy distraction for Dad. While Dad was never able to come see me lift or compete in person, he did catch it on a competition videotape.

Before I knew it, I was 23 years old, walking down the aisle to marry the best and only workout partner I had ever had. Some of the guys from the gym were there with their wives. We took a group photo with everyone flexing. Our adult lives were taking off. I was working hard as a copywriter at an in-house creative department for a major publisher. That was 8–10 hours of my day. After work, Craig and I would meet at the gym where we'd train with our gym friends for a few hours. More hard work, but a different kind. It was our happy hour. Then, we'd head home for a chicken and pasta concoction, and some favorite TV shows like *Seinfeld, Friends,* and *NYPD Blue.* Then finally off to bed to wake up refreshed enough to do it all over again the next day.

The other powerlifters were becoming some of our closest friends. They cheered me on to keep pushing, to keep loading more weight on the bar. They always believed in me, even on days when I didn't. While I loved powerlifting with the guys and having an athletic connection with a competitive team where I actually felt like I belonged, I had a secret interest in what some of the other people in the gym were up to.

The bodybuilders.

THE BODYBUILDING YEARS

The bodybuilders brought me back to the *David* statue, to Uncle Steve, and Dad in his mind's eye. To beautiful, statuesque works of art, and my love of drawing figures such as the ones I was influenced by as a child. My artistic eye appreciated the lines and aesthetics of the human form, the muscle shapes and fullness, and how the different muscle groups joined together.

I began my field work in the investigation of what it meant to be a bodybuilder. I did a lot of observation in the gym, as well as book and magazine reading. One thing that stood out immediately was how much bodybuilders tuned the world out. They wore Walkmans, which were the first personal music devices, that piped music in their ears so loud that I could hear the song thumps just by standing near them. Whether they were female or male, young or old, short or tall, bodybuilders seemed to all have a singular, inward focus. I was naturally an introspective type, always had been. Even with their training partners standing right next to them, there was no talking, no high-fiving, no cheering each other on. You just did your lifting. A regime that was clearly methodical and precise. No wavering from a plan or getting distracted by outside forces or other gym members. Bodybuilders were driven.

Little by little, I began to supplement my powerlifting workouts with bodybuilding exercises. When I'd head over to a cable crossover machine after benching to further work and refine my pecs, the guys would tease me. To my powerlifting buddies, bodybuilders were "cushy" and narcissistic. The anti-hardcore. I accepted their ribbing, laughed it off, and went to work anyway.

Squats, benches, and deadlifts began to get peppered with other, more fine-tuning exercises such as dumbbell flies to shape the inner pectoralis major, concentration curls for the main heads of the biceps, toe raises with angled foot positions to hit the calves differently (toes in for the outer calves, toes out for the inner calves), and tons of abdominal work. I did this for a few weeks. Little boxes were beginning to form on my stomach; for the first time, I was developing a six-pack. I started experimenting with tightening my diet, which included more fresh vegetables and grilled chicken, and way fewer foods made with white flour or chemicals I couldn't pronounce. The massive bowls of pasta Craig and I climbed into each night were replaced with a medley of brown rice, vegetables, and chicken. I was adding more cardio fitness to burn calories and lose fat. I was also reading a lot about the sport, from magazines such as *Flex* and *Muscle and Fitness* to books including Bill Pearl's *Keys to the Inner Universe,* a 600-plus-page bodybuilding bible of exercises. The muscles I had spent years building up through powerlifting were getting further refined by bodybuilding.

Compete.

My inner voice was pestering me again to reach for something I never tried before. I began to shift my workouts even more. I already had well-established back muscles, bicep peaks, and quad sweeps from beast-mode lifting for the last few years. I had developed a "Christmas tree" back where the muscle striations looked like the tapered shape of a holiday tree. Now, I was learning how to refine those muscles, to add to or take away shape and size for an overall aesthetic. With powerlifting, my lifts were heavy, and the reps were lower, which were great for building a muscular foundation and developing strength. With bodybuilding, I lightened the pounds to perform more repetitions. More reps helped to chisel and refine each muscle group. Sets with 50 reps at a time put me on the verge of tears because it hurt like crazy. These were "to failure" sets. But what exactly *is* failure? My mind locking in on a number and reaching that number with my body? My body giving up from pushing it as far as it could at that moment in time? Both. I also added cardio to my daily workouts to start losing weight to achieve a ripped effect. Diet was critical like never before.

I signed up for my first bodybuilding competition. Drug-free was still my personal approach to lifting, so I entered an ANPPC (All-Natural Physique and Power Conference) bodybuilding show in Tarrytown, New York. Once again, ignorance worked in my favor. I had no idea what grueling felt like…what true physical pain felt like…what it meant to literally be brought to tears from exercise…what head games could do to an athlete…until I trained for bodybuilding. All I knew was that I was setting a behemoth goal for myself and I couldn't wait to get started.

Typically, I would enter a show that was a few months away, which would give me plenty of time to strategize a 16-week training program. Four months of training that got harder and harder as time went on. It wasn't just the work in the gym anymore; bodybuilding was a lifestyle. From the meals to the posing practice, both of which get more intense as you get closer to the big day, bodybuilding consumed me.

Preparing for bodybuilding was like being in a crockpot for weeks. Low and slow at first, as I added more training and minor adjustments to an already clean diet. This was as basic as cutting out refined sugars or cream in coffee. But with each passing week, the heat got turned up on the cooker. Workouts got longer and more frequent until I was training twice a day for over two hours each time. The diet got tighter and stricter until all I was eating was egg whites, grilled chicken, steamed broccoli, and baked potatoes. We bought pallets of eggs, not dozens, each week. Mostly, we boiled them to be able to quickly down four or five egg whites at a time for much-needed protein. I'd mash the whites, slice them, halve them, warm them, throw them in shakes and salads—anything I could do to simulate variety.

I scheduled everything, from workouts that meshed with corporate responsibilities to meals when attending special occasions centered around food. Preparation was at the forefront of everything I did. Meals got packed the night before just in case I couldn't order something at an office lunch *dry and plain* off the menu. With each day or week that I'd "X" off the calendar, bringing me one step closer to the day of competition, I would feel my personal power swelling. The harder it all got, the stronger I felt. The deeper I dove into each week, the more invested I became in my process. Low-impact cardio workouts, which were better for maintaining muscle and burning fat, increased in time and frequency. I'd walk outside at lunch to burn off extra calories or sneak into a conference room to practice my posing for 10–15 minutes.

Posing was part dance, part standing still as the *David* statue. It was what you did to best showcase your muscles on the day of the competition. Posing is exactly what it sounds like; when you compete in bodybuilding, you perform a host of mandatory poses that exemplify your muscularity. These are the following: quarter turns, front double biceps, rear double biceps, front lat spread, rear lat spread, side chest, side triceps, and front abdominals and thighs. It sounds pretty simple; it's not. One inch too much one way or the slightest misalignment of a hand position could completely alter how your muscles were showcased. A wide sweep of the latissimus could collapse if your hands were held too high on your waist during a lat spread. Quadriceps received the highest scores when you could make the striations in your sweep stand out. This came from a skillfully placed and properly flexed foot on the floor. The boxes in your abs didn't look as sharp unless you hit the precise point of flexion.

And then there was the challenge of *holding* the poses. Flexing muscles as hard as possible for 20–30 minutes, while on stage under hot lights, and not making a straining poop face, is close to impossible. All that, and you need to smile. The judges give you points, as well as take away points, for muscularity, symmetry, and hardness. Like chess pieces on a board, you and your competition get moved around the stage based on the judges' requests. Move here, stand next to her, come in front, go in back. This shuffling of bodies helps the judges see you, side by side, against the others. You start to feel like cattle, especially because they call you out by the number on the tag you pinned to the bottom of your posing suit. If your number got called in the first round, it was a good thing: your physique stood out. Typically, these are the competitors who take top placements at the end of the evening show. The others get ranked in order from best to "worst" until the judges determine *last place*. Coming in 15th out of 15 competitors is crushing to the ego.

A competition has two parts: (1) the day show when the judges scrutinize your physique against the other competitors and (2) the night show when things get more entertaining for the audience with music and posing routines, although there still is extensive judging involved.

If you do well in the day, you typically do well in the night. There's also the chance that you flatten out by nighttime, which can happen from the carb depletion/carb load process going awry, plus basic dehydration. But if you can hold onto what you've worked so hard for, you just might walk away with a trophy. The "holding on" part is a bit of a crapshoot at this point. Eating the right foods in between the morning and evening events and keeping the water intake low enough so you don't smooth out, yet not so low that you wilt away, can make a difference. On a regular day, I bloated easily, so I had to be extra careful. Without water in the muscles, they can flatten out. Carb depleting the last few days before competition, which always made me mentally loopy, needed to be topped off by carb loading right up until the day of the show. That could include eating foods such as baked potatoes, peanut butter, and even small bits of cake or chocolate (high sugar content) to help quickly pull water back into the muscles. This makes the muscles look plump and full. Some competitors would even drink wine right before going on stage to help with vascularity.

The morning after I had my "celebratory" meal after a show (it was always at the diner for a cheeseburger, fries and a milkshake—carbs and sugar, galore), my body was always more ripped and vascular than during the competition the day before. It was freaky! But I never had the courage to actually eat a *Snickers* bar before I walked on a stage. It felt too risky; after so many months of hard work, I was too afraid I'd smooth out right there in front of the judges.

For the night show, the spectators arrive, the competitors do their individual posing routines, and the final winners are announced. My dance background came in handy for the posing routine. In my first competition, I choreographed a routine to George Thorogood's "Bad to the Bone." Ninety seconds long, it had to include mandatory poses, plus any other creative movements of my choice to highlight my muscularity. The "most muscular" was my go-to pose because it seemed to showcase my strengths, such as shoulders and chest. The individual posing routines can get the crowd just as pumped as the athlete, as evidenced by screams and cheers. At the night show, you're typically depleted beyond belief, and because you've been flexing as hard as possible all day, you tend to cramp up. Flexing is what you do to make your muscles stand out.

In my beginning stages of bodybuilding, I competed in local events, choosing those in the tristate area. It was easier and more cost-effective to drive to the venue on a Friday afternoon and stay at a hotel for one night until the day of competition, which usually fell on a Saturday inside a high school auditorium. But as I became more competitive in the sport, I took road trips with Craig to places such as Washington, DC and South Carolina. The stakes got higher and the competition fiercer. If I was going to be serious about this sport, no decision was to be made on convenience.

In powerlifting, you either lift the weight, or you don't. Judges call the lift good or not. You can be standing on the platform and if you drop the weight or your knees buckle, then, oh well, better luck next time. While you may be competing against other lifters, you are in constant battle against your own "PRs." Conversely, competitive bodybuilding is a completely subjective sport where it's you against everyone else.

Bodybuilders are at the mercy of a judge's opinion and personal preference of what a physique should look like on that particular day. Yes, there are judging criteria like symmetry, muscularity, and vascularity, but what looks pleasing to one judge may not to another. Beauty is most definitely in the eye of the beholder. If you win or place in the top five, then none of this is an issue. When you don't do well and wonder what just happened after killing yourself the last four months, you can get a little disgruntled. And with carbohydrate depletion making it hard to produce clear thoughts, you can get emotional. Every competitor wants to win, or place, and, if the athletes are all in prime shape, you never know who is going to take the title. There is way less comradery in the pump-up room, which is the place backstage where competitors flush their veins with blood from quick curls and rope pulls. You want to be more pumped than the next guy before you get on stage. More oiled up. More ready to kick some serious competitive butt.

Still, with all that tumult, I was hooked. Probably even more so, I was loving the process leading up to the event: the weeks and weeks of pushing to the max, the transformation of my body, the goals and my unwavering commitment to them, and the educating of self to learn more about things like carb depletion. Carbs hold water. If you don't eat them, then you hold less water. If you're smooth (holding water), you can't see your muscle definition. If you're ripped (not holding water), then you're on top of the world because your skin looks paper thin and everything underneath it (muscle striations and veins) pops. In a bodybuilding competition, coming in smooth is the kiss of death. A coworker once looked at my pictures a few days after a competition, one where I hadn't done well. "Look at all these girls' legs. They're all bumpy. Yours are all smooth and nice." I wanted to cry.

You want to have the widest shoulders, a back flair like a python, quadriceps that sweep, biceps that peak, and abs of the six-pack kind. And if the bodybuilding gods are working with you, you are not a few days from getting your period and experiencing bloat. Some women drop their body fat so low that they no longer menstruate.

Competitive bodybuilding required that I be on stage, under hot lights, in front of a panel of judges and a host of spectators, in a posing suit, which was basically a bikini. I had a friend in high school who entered a bikini contest and I thought how that was something I would *never* do. Yet, here I was, in two small pieces of Lycra, and strutting across a stage showing off my body. But, for me, the difference was nature versus nurture. I never had one of those bodies that people would ogle over at the beach. Mine represented a culmination of hard work, sweat, reps, and unwavering determination. I was damn proud of that.

Bodybuilders need to be tan when they compete. Under the stark stage lights, tanned skin creates a more dramatic look, showcasing better contrast for muscles to stand out. Getting a tan in the middle of March was a challenge if you lived in the tristate area. For two weeks before a show, I'd snooze in tanning beds that cooked my skin until I could smell it. The hard-shell plastic goggles covered my eyes from the blue glow coming from the panini-type cooker. The ritual the night before a competition included applying liquid bronzer over my entire body to ensure a deep, tan glow. It was a special kind made for bodybuilders. It smelled terrible and went on looking very burnt orange. Proper application was critical because you could easily wind up with streaks and patches of dark brown around your elbows and knees. Craig painted me with a small sponge brush from Home Depot while I stood naked on a towel. Then I'd stand there for 20 minutes to dry. And, of course, I was always standing under a drafty vent. In the morning, a light shower rinsed off any excess goop. It was a ridiculous ritual but a necessary evil to achieve the perfect complexion for the competition stage. The final layer of artistry was applied right before hitting the stage—a coat of baby oil. Or cooking spray applied straight from the can. Not too much that I'd appear greasy, but just enough to be shiny. I looked (and often smelled) like a rotisserie chicken.

Competition was a two-part process: (1) the rigorous, 16-week long training cycle where I put my heart and soul into creating the best version of me and (2) the day of competition, when I stood on stage to present the culmination of the many months of hard work.

When going out to dinner in the weeks prior to competition, I would repeat my order to the waiter, emphasizing the key words: grilled chicken breast *plain. Steamed* broccoli. Wheat toast *dry*. When a rare bowl of pasta was ordered and came out glistening, I would say, "This pasta looks shiny. Is there oil on it?" My refrigerator was void of fats, sweets, alcohol—anything that would negatively affect my training. Luckily, Craig was just as willing to join the mania, even though he wasn't competing. It made it that much easier to forge ahead without guilt of being an absolute bore.

I was the girl who brought stinky lunches to work. It was an open work space with cubbies, so, as soon as I cracked open my Tupperware, my colleagues would rag on me. The scent of hard-boiled eggs, broccoli, and trout, all in one bowl, was stifling. But my coworkers' teasing was all in good fun because they knew I was on a mission, and they were witnesses to my physical transformation. They always had questions: "How long are your workouts? Can I see your abs?" They were so supportive, many of them coming to see me compete.

One day, while explaining my crazy bodybuilding lifestyle to a group of coworkers, simultaneously digging into a container of steamed fish and spinach, I said, "I guess I'm living up to my nickname, HercuLisa." It just popped out. No one looked at me with a that's-so-dumb face. In fact, their expressions solidified how much it made sense. HercuLisa equaled strength. The kind that I was building on the outside and, even more, cultivating on the inside.

Spring was the main competitive season. I'd find myself saying farewell to my favorite foods right after the December holidays. The more often I competed, the deeper the pit in my stomach grew because, as a seasoned competitor, I knew what kind of pain and the depth of the personal tests I would have to endure. The closer I came to my competition date, the harder things got. On Mondays, I knew I was about to face the bar and squat. Leg press sets went from 15 reps per set to 50. Cardio sessions extended from 30 minutes each time to an hour. Abs snowballed from 200 reps per session to 500. As much as I was torturing myself through competitive bodybuilding, I was also testing my personal boundaries. Not just with muscle, but with mind. *How strong are you? How much stronger can you be? How much can you take?* Training for competition was about me pushing me.

On the day of competition, I always wore a hooded zipper sweatshirt and baggy sweats over my posing suit. The zipper made for easy on and off without messing up my tan and makeup. Pulling the hood up over my hair-sprayed coif, which was usually pulled into a tight bun, added to a feeling of going within a cocoon of strength. The energy backstage made my pulse race as dozens of other women and I pumped up. Push-ups, towel tugs, bicep curls—everything to get the blood pumping inside the veins that were popping out of my skin. And if they weren't visibly popping, I hadn't carb depleted and carb reloaded enough. But I couldn't entertain any head games at that point. *You did your best.* The feeling inside was of power and excitement, of being on top of the world, yet scared that I was about to get toppled by the competition.

The moment you walk onto the stage, you become a number, a category, a physique. Your inner fire and the integrity you've held to give 110 percent 24/7 for these last 16 weeks—heck, these past five years—can only be measured by the body standing in front of the row of blazer-clad men and women in the judges' pit. You dare not make eye contact because they don't want to see you; they just need to look at you. Instead, you look out into the dark auditorium to find a distant point in the atmosphere. A wall clock like the one they used to have in the school cafeteria. The silhouette of someone's head that you imagine is a supportive friend. *Focus on one thing. Like that EXIT sign. How many words can you make from it? Ex. Tie. Tex. It.* Or if you can't find anything fast enough, you dig into your mental image bank and lock in on something. A place. A memory. A face.

The announcer calls your class—short or tall, lightweight or heavyweight. You'd better remember your personal number, 21 or 2 or 40 depending upon how many people entered the contest, because this is the only way that'll you know when the judges are addressing you in the lineup. That number is written in Sharpie marker on a round cardboard tag that's hanging by a safety pin that you pricked into the Lycra of your posing suit. A suit that you paid too much money for because they don't sell these off the rack at Macy's, so you had one custom made. Actually, two, in case something ripped or got stained by the bronzer. They're not bathing suits; they're posing suits. And they have to sit just right in all the right places. They're designed for moving when you do, not for lying on the beach. The only thing you want popping out are your veins and muscles. You're wearing either hot pink, deep red, or basic black.

You're practically naked. You're barefoot and the hardwood stage floor is filthy. The stage lights beat down on you and you sweat like a hog because you're also posing your heart out. Posing that way takes every ounce of your remaining strength. You're grateful to be sweating because that means the last drops of water are leaving your body. A close to dehydrated body equals a ripped physique. As you sweat, you worry that your spray tan is running and that your makeup is melting. There's a bead of sweat trailing down your face, but you don't dare wipe it away. You need to hold your composure. No fidgeting or fixing. You pretend you're a beautiful, well-crafted statue. *David.*

And you smile.

A constant, frozen, face-hurting smile because it's all about aesthetics, and what judge wants to give points to a sourpuss competitor? Your mouth is so dry from lack of water that your top lip is sticking to your teeth. You wonder if you should have smeared Vaseline on your incisors like you read about in one of the magazines.

You think you need to pee, but you're just nervous. You're too dehydrated to pee.

You think about food. Food. Food. Food. About the meal you want to have when this is all done tonight. You'll either be celebrating or wallowing. Either way, something greasy and drippy. Something that you've deprived yourself of for so long that all you do is dream about it. A burger and fries. Pizza. Chocolate chip muffins. Milkshakes. You crave food from the movie *Grease.* Oh yeah, grease. You're a hungry wolf, yet so physically, mentally, and emotionally drained you could curl up behind that velvet curtain you just walked out from and call it a day. But you won't because this is the moment you've been training for. You squeeze your muscles just a little tighter, lick your dry lips, and flex your heart out. You move all the mental crap aside and focus. You swap out every morsel of thought to enter a void of nothing.

Nothing can stop you now.

You feed off the cheering crowd and you hear your people calling your name, not your number. Their screams are the cardiac paddles you need to keep you alive up there. You tell yourself *Don't let go, hang in there, you got this.* When the judging is done and the announcer thanks your class and asks you to leave the stage, you gladly walk off, feeling like you just swam the Atlantic.

For the years that I was a competitive bodybuilder, I threw myself completely into the most challenging, solitary, exhilarating sport of my life. It taught me just how hungry I could be. Literally and figuratively. It wasn't enough anymore that my max effort went to the weights; to succeed in this training cycle I had to create a 365-day program that basically consumed my life. I won a few titles here and there, including Best Poser in my first competition (I guess my dance experience did come in handy), and one win which qualified me to compete as a professional bodybuilder. I achieved the status of pro bodybuilder, which is hilarious to me, the girl who ate cupcakes during gym class. Pro is just fancy talk for "competing for money." First place winners could snag one or two thousand dollars, while fifth place might get three hundred dollars. Just enough money to cover your hotel, meals, and gas. Once I turned pro, I only competed in professional events. As long as I never actually took home prize money (which I never did), I could continue to compete in the amateurs. But it felt like reverse progress, so I didn't.

The pro competitions I partook in were all drug-free, drug-tested events. More peeing in cups and I even had to take a lie detector test once to prove my steroid-free status. I was so carb depleted and dehydrated that I almost passed out.

The level of competition was incredible in the pros. These women were seasoned, many of them training for more than a decade, and with muscularity, rippedness, and symmetry like I had never seen before in person. I had to up my game. Heavier weights, more sets, longer cardio sessions, extra posing, a tighter diet. Smarter training that required more reading and more experimentation, such as swapping out dumbbell press for bench press in hopes of keeping my neck injuries from flaring up. Or planning my dieting cycle so that I would "peak" (carb deplete and then carb load) at precisely the right moment, which was the day of the show.

My body, however, was not on board like it was even a year prior. Just because I kept training harder and harder didn't mean that I was getting better. In fact, it was quite the opposite. My muscles were always tired, I was constantly getting tweaked, and I'd often get a stiff neck for days after a heavy chest workout. I could barely turn my head to drive. My body was less responsive than it used to be, which was evident in my slower gains. I was always craving something I wouldn't allow myself to eat. Even with my body feeling like it wanted to tap out, my mind would not have it. So, I pressed on.

I pushed through pain and doubt, struggle and insecurity, frustration and fear that everything I worked so hard for would just crumble. I awakened at 5 am to work out before going to the office. I ate only the foods that were bodybuilding "sanctioned" items (yes, chicken breast, rice, steamed broccoli). I kept up with my workout journals, charting everything I did in and out of the gym. I strategized the year ahead to the precise date of my next competition. But for the first time in years, I could see my body rebelling. However, while my physical strength was rolling in ebbs and flows, my mind was on fire. With my body breaking down at times, it was becoming that much more evident how strong my mind had to be. How strong it could be.

In between being a competitive pro bodybuilder, I was also just a regular 25-year-old starting out her adult life. Everything was new: my full-time job as a copywriter (no longer a junior writer); my marriage; my apartment in Bayside, Queens; my shiny, techy, totally beautiful word processor. It was a wedding gift from Craig; up until then, I had been writing long-hand or on an electric typewriter. It was on this machine that I began to do some of my best writing yet.

One Sunday afternoon, as I perused *The New York Times* classified section for fun, an ad for a freelance writer caught my eye. The description might as well have been written for me. It said something like: "New national magazine looking for a freelance writer, with 2–3 years of experience, to write a monthly column about fitness books and videos; knowledge of bodybuilding and fitness a plus." I was already employed as a publishing copywriter in the creative department at Doubleday Book & Music Clubs in Garden City, Long Island. But this opportunity was too perfect for me to ignore. Plus, freelance. I could do that plus my regular job.

I typed up a long cover letter explaining why I was the person for the job, both professionally and personally. A manifesto. I attached my resume along with one or two writing samples (I didn't have much yet) and a list of my competitive bodybuilding experiences and dropped the entire package in the mail. Just like every other test I had given myself these last few years, I had this strong, probably unfounded belief that I could "win" the job. I believed in myself.

A week later, the phone rang. It was the editor-in-chief of the magazine. She was preparing the launch and was interested in me as a contributing writer. I was bursting with excitement! We scheduled a face-to-face meeting at her office in Connecticut. We hit it off and I got the job! The editor was a wonderful mentor to me, plus a really kind person. She treated me as if I was a seasoned professional even though I was just starting out on all fronts. Suddenly, I was a monthly columnist for a new magazine called *Bodybuilding Lifestyles*. The magazine offered an impressive line-up of celebrity bodybuilders and was backed by the WBF (World Bodybuilding Federation), which was part of the WWF (World Wrestling Federation) at the time. There was a lot of corporate brawn behind this launch. Part of the mission of the magazine, in addition to the bodybuilding tips and information, was to showcase certain bodybuilders as superstars, just like it was done in wrestling.

Aside from being a blast of an experience, as well as an income booster, being the monthly columnist for *Bodybuilding Lifestyles* fortified my personal growth. The role:

1.   Validated me as a writer;

2.   Validated me as a bodybuilder;

3.   Came with cool perks.

The first fortification came at a time when I was building my self-esteem in my profession. My corporate work was creative and challenging, and I was soaking in every experience from anyone who would share expertise. But being given a column to write each month was a different level of responsibility that I couldn't wait to take on. Someone trusted me, believed in me.

I was also in my peak competitive bodybuilding years, now in the ranks of professional bodybuilding, despite starting to feel the effects of burnout. Nothing looked better than seeing my byline on paper or hearing a show's announcer: "Lisa Safran is a professional writer and a competitive bodybuilder...blah, blah, blah." I was in my sweet spot—it was my first life experience where my two budding passions intersected.

Each month, boxes of books sent directly from publishers would arrive at my home for me to read and review. The topics were on everything from bodybuilding workouts to diets to personal life stories. Sometimes, the column had to include multiple books, so I was tasked with creating an overall theme. I interviewed iconic bodybuilders like Carla Dunlap, who was the winner of the 1983 Ms. Olympia, the most coveted female bodybuilding competition. I got exercise videotapes to test out before anyone else could buy them. I even received a pair of inline skates as a piece of "cardio equipment" to test and keep. When the weather turned nice, a few of my friends at work brought their skates to the office, and we skated around the parking lot during lunch. It was socializing, research, and fitness all rolled up into one.

I was given a press pass to an event at the WWF headquarters in Connecticut. It was a bodybuilding forum to stimulate a buzz around the magazine and the WBF in general, which was preparing to launch its own competitions. It was a who's who of famous bodybuilders and workout legends—Tom Platz, Fred Hatfield, the Quinn brothers, just to name a few. Of course, I brought my workout partner with me, and together we drooled over all the "stars." We took pictures with celebs like star-struck kids, but I had to remind myself that I was "press." So, technically, I was on the inside and I needed to behave as such. Tom Platz, also known as "Quadzilla," did a squatting event to see how many reps he could get with a hefty weight. I think it was 315 pounds on the bar. After he pounded out 50 reps, he racked the weight and staggered away from the bar. Somehow, I was suddenly hugging Tom Platz. Craig was not the least bit jealous. In fact, I was his hero for a very long time. I had hugged Quadzilla!

My columnist writing gig lasted less than two years (the magazine eventually folded), but it was probably two of the most exciting years of my writing career. There was connectivity between what I did in and out of work, who I was, and what I wanted to be. I was finding my voice as a writer through the lens of fitness.

The writing experience from *Bodybuilding Lifestyles* became the springboard for future writing assignments with other fitness magazines including *Female Bodybuilding, Natural Physique, Energy for Women,* and *Fit Pregnancy.* Whether I was writing personal essays such as "Notes from the Road: All Powered Up and Completely Snowed In" (it was about a powerlifting meet I competed in in Wilkes Barre, Pennsylvania and how we got stuck there for a few days because of a bad storm) or interviewing other female lifters in an article called "Women in Power," I continued to expand as both a writer and a bodybuilder.

One of my favorite articles was "California Pumpin': The Bodybuilder's Guide to Sightseeing in Southern California," which appeared in *Female Bodybuilding.* It chronicled our week-long vacation to California that was built around visiting all the famous gyms. Craig and I meticulously planned out each day, making sure that we hit every hot spot on the West Coast including Gold's Gym (one in San Diego, then another in Venice), World Gym, and Venice Beach aka Muscle Beach. We spotted tons of professional bodybuilders, picked up lifting tips just by watching them, and mostly glommed off the energy of being in an area known as the "mecca of bodybuilding." Most of our friends were using their vacation time to break from the normal routine; Craig and I used ours to amplify it.

The connectivity between competition and what sells magazines became more evident to me. I became more in tune with the press coverage from various bodybuilding magazines at my pro competitions. Photographers and reporters were present at events, tasked with getting the stories that would sell magazines. It was suddenly evident to me as to who they were told to watch, and who was irrelevant. At first, I was part of a "rookie to watch" category, which resulted in a short profile on me in one of the magazines. That pushed me to train more and compete more, going from one show to the next without real rest periods in between. I was constantly training, but, unfortunately, placing lower and lower each time I got back on the stage. This rookie to watch was burning out.

As I placed lower and lower in the competitive line-ups, I grew less enamored with the sport. My body hurt. I was tired. My mind was wandering.

And then, out of nowhere, Dad died. He took a nap one afternoon, right in the very bed that he sat on to do bicep curls years ago, and never woke up.

In between helping my mother, whose Parkinson's was progressing, adjust to life without Dad, and grappling with my own loss, I made a personal declaration that I was ready to officially retire from competitive bodybuilding.

There was no anger or remorse or guilt. I did not feel as if I had quit on myself like when I ran track or danced. I wasn't sprinting away from something or avoiding the hard work. Bodybuilding competition and I had a great run. It was just time. I never felt stronger in my decision. Leaving the competitive stage didn't mean that I left the gym. In fact, I jumped back into my workouts with full force. Just training the way I had when I first started. I wasn't training for competition anymore; I was training for Dad. For all the exercises he couldn't do these last few years, because he was too defeated. For the many muscles he sketched with pen over an old photo of himself to capture his bodybuilder's dream bod. For the dumbbells he gave me when all I wanted was a party.

Losing a parent without gearing up for it is like tearing a muscle that you counted on every single day. Pop, and there it goes. Curls right up into a funny-shaped ball that leaves you black and blue for weeks. Maybe it needs surgical reattachment. Maybe it will heal on its own but will hurt for the rest of your life. There's just no way of knowing. But just like it does for training muscles, pain can lead you toward greater refinement. It just takes time. I had to believe that to press on.

By now, Craig and I had established a solid reputation as the "iron" couple. Our other married friends had distinct compartments to their lives—one in and one out of the gym. For us, working out permeated everything. At the gym, it was all about the guys. The wives did their exercise elsewhere at places that offered group fitness classes because they feared getting bulky from weight training. So, our daily gym conversations were about workouts—goals, gains, disappointments, that kind of banter—not around adult topics such as mortgages and career paths. The only time we talked about work or family was during warm-ups before the serious training began. As we primed our rotator cuffs for benching or stretched out our "hammies" for deadlifts, someone would mention how the first trimester was going or share about something cute that baby Paul was doing.

While the gym posse could easily slip into gym talk, even when we weren't in the gym, the wives were great about bringing the conversation back to other topics. Otherwise, we were always talking about the time someone blew out his bench shirt or when I accidentally clipped Pete's nose between two dumbbells while he was spotting me. When we did all get together outside of the gym, either for dinner or a BBQ, it would then become evident to me and Craig that plans for having future gym rats were happening all around us.

Why weren't we?

Because, when we were at the gym, we were happily tucked inside a time capsule/comfort zone with the same cast of characters, same workouts, same worn-to-perfection gray sweats, same pump-up music, same inside jokes, and then the same buckwheat pancakes with egg whites at IHOP every Saturday morning after a killer workout. It was an odd mix of personal growth and being stuck in exactly the same place where we started 10 years ago. It was during this time that we took an honest look at our own lives and goals outside of the gym. Craig and I made the decision to start building a family.

We approached getting pregnant with a casual, "when it happens, it'll happen" mindset. This carefree spirit was freeing and fun. However, I secretly struggled with the notion that my body was about to transform in ways that were completely out of my control. I was stuck between the pull of wanting to have a baby, feeling overwhelmed with letting go of a 10-year-long fitness discipline, being afraid of becoming a mom, and being even more terrified that I would never have the opportunity to be one.

When we didn't hit our "goal" on the first few attempts at pregnancy, I shifted my focus toward working out the only way I knew how, with intensity. Maybe I wasn't quite ready for this life change, and the Universe stepped in on my behalf by making conception tricky. But, over the next year, the challenge of getting pregnant was starting to look like it was unattainable. Unlike choosing a competition or mapping out a 16-week workout cycle, we couldn't circle a date on the calendar and say, "Yup, that's a good time to get pregnant." Conception didn't care what we wanted or when, or how hard I was willing to work at it.

When turned to *if* as I entered the most trying phase of my life. Trying to get pregnant, trying to pull back from the intensity of working out, trying to let go of the desire to get back on a stage or platform and do better than my last competition. Trying to figure out who I was at this moment in my life. A retired competitive bodybuilder? A fitness fanatic who was about to hit the pause button on her obsession? A woman who wants to have a baby but can't? A daughter who lost her dad and whose mom was getting sicker? I was mentally and emotionally drained.

We struggled with fertility issues for a few years. We tried going on carefree vacations or weekend getaways because people were always telling us to "stop thinking about it so much and it will happen." Not true for us. Eventually, we sought out a fertility specialist. Experts say you need a full year of unsuccessful attempts at conception in order to fit the infertility criteria. But, as time ticked on, we felt the pressure of defeat. One year of failure (that's the word that fit the feeling) rolled into two years. These years were the antithesis of the body control I had perfected in the prior decade. No extra sweat or reps or hours in the gym could alter our predicament.

Yet getting pregnant was all about my body—a body I had grown used to manipulating. For nearly 10 years, it allowed me to shape and mold it, to ignore its pain, to make it do what I wanted it to, and then to "perform" on the culminating day of competition. Suddenly, I felt as if my body had turned on me. My stress was off the charts. I would cry like a baby when a TV show was interrupted by a car commercial with a family in it. (Hormone treatments only made it worse.) I broke out in head-to-toe hives and my best friend, Maria, brought me Aveeno oatmeal to bathe in. My number one stress reliever—intense, butt-kicking exercise—was no longer on the table. I was like a can of effervescent soda, having been shaken vigorously, trapped inside with a broken pull tab.

I had given up all rigorous training out of fear that I would do something to hurt my body. Cinching a weightlifting belt around my waist had to be bad for my reproductive organs. Lifting too heavy was a sure-fire way to injure some key body part. Too much cardio made my heart rate spike too high, which all the books advised against. Without the physical outlet to work through my frustration, I didn't know where to channel my energy. I puttered a lot. I got back to journaling. I still went to the gym a few times a week, but instead I grabbed lightweight dumbbells and did a lot of light walking on the treadmill, light cardio, light stretching. Emphasis on *light*. Recreational fitness felt like munching on carrot sticks when I hadn't eaten in a week. My mind was fully committed to pushing myself like I always did, but this time I had to push to be still.

You can be comfortable with uncomfortable.

My mind was taking over more than ever, training my body to not instinctually step in with hard, pounding work. My thoughts were all over the place, yet it was my head that needed to keep me from losing it.

With the help of medical miracles and an abundance of hope, we eventually got pregnant. We were ecstatic but petrified. Afraid that something would go wrong, or that it was all too good to be true. I wanted to white-knuckle my way through the next few months, afraid to breathe the wrong way and hurt the baby, and also to brace myself to surrender to something I had very little control over.

With bodybuilding, control over the physical self is at the core of everything you do. I felt very stuck between worlds: happiness in finally being pregnant and secretly frustrated by how much my body was not mine anymore. And then, of course, came a steaming plate of guilt for even thinking this way.

I was used to daily muscle soreness. I actually looked forward to it because it was a tangible validation that I had worked hard the day before. The cause and effect manifested through my physical being in such clear and measurable ways. Without the pain, I wondered if I worked hard enough. Pregnancy, however, opened up opportunities for my body to speak to me in different ways. I just needed to train myself to listen. My childhood years presented a disconnect with my body unless I was feeling pain from a skinned knee or a charley horse. I never paid much mind to the parts underneath the flesh—the organs, cells, DNA, muscle. These were things I couldn't see. Only through diet and exercise, like the strict regimen I followed before a bodybuilding competition, would some of the inside stuff be revealed via my exterior layer. Muscle fibers and striations, pumped-up veins, bones. But again, these were tangible.

The first trimester, the time when you don't actually look pregnant, but you feel very different, helped me to start listening to my body. Well, maybe I wasn't fully listening but at least not ignoring it when it was crying out for certain foods or rest. Those first few weeks all I craved was food at the pizzeria. Chicken parm, meatball subs, pizza, baked ziti—anything where a suspension of cheese hung from fork to mouth. The vats of red sauce and salt satiated my inner *Goodfellas*. For the past decade, I rarely ate these things because I was preparing for some show or meet. Suddenly, it was all I craved, so I honored that and ate it.

The workout partner who always encouraged me to do more, lift more, push more was treating me as if I were made of porcelain. "Take it easy," he said. *Easy? How do I do that?* This is when I accidentally discovered something I had snubbed my nose at for years: yoga.

For me, hardcore weight training was the exact opposite of yoga, which would have been the precise reason to incorporate it, but I wasn't that evolved yet. Instead, I viewed yoga as the lesser choice. The wimpy way. If there were five nights in a week that I could exercise, I was going to invest each of those nights at the gym, not on some yoga mat. My only exposure to yoga had been in Florida when I was a little girl.

Grandma taught a yoga class to seniors at her adult community and, while sitting on my pool towel in the rec room trying to reach my toes, I'd watch all the older ladies stick their tongues way out and roar. Then they would stand on all fours while Grandma talked gibberish about imagined places and breathing. All they cared about was breathing. I was always amazed by how you could open your mouth wide, breathe into your hand, and discover that the air was warm. A second later, you could purse your lips, breathe into that same hand, and feel that the air was cool. I was already breathing just fine; I didn't understand all the fuss. However, it was fun to hear Grandma tell people to act like lions and dogs, and they would! And then we'd get ice cream sandwiches at the clubhouse after class.

My other yoga exposure was through my Uncle Steve and Aunt Ladene; they were the real yoga pioneers in our family because they had their own local television show called *Stretch & Flex*. It taught viewers how to move their bodies in therapeutic ways. Together, they would demonstrate the poses while Uncle Steve explained the benefits. Aunt Ladene's super-long braid would hang down sideways as she formed triangle pose (*Trikonasana*) with her arms and legs. I was mesmerized by how the tip of her braid grazed the floor. I imagined it to be a Tarzan rope that I could hold onto and swing from place to place.

Flash forward 25 years to me in my first trimester, attending the mindfulness/meditation class offered at my local hospital. The nurses suggested it as a stress management tool while going through fertility treatments and the early stages of my pregnancy. At this point, I was open to trying anything to help with my stress.

In the first class, I was instantly smitten with a meditation technique called "The Relaxation Response." From a book by Dr. Herbert Benson, it basically outlined a guided mind-body approach to relaxation. This felt like the opposite of the "fight or flight" response to everything I had trained my body to do. In one particular class, the instructor handed out oranges: "Close your eyes. Hold your orange and feel the rippling skin. Begin to peel it. Smell the pungent sweetness. Taste the juiciness of each section; chew each piece slowly and thoughtfully. Imagine it flowing down your throat. Be one with your fruit."

Be one with your fruit.

I mulled that over in my mind. With my eyes shut, my ears were that much more in tune with the sounds of peel breaking, of juice piercing the air, of people chewing and some snickering, and of breathing. I was used to the sound of panting breaths during a killer cardio workout. I had never stopped to notice the soft, rhythmic, calming sounds of normal breath. The kind I'd been doing every day since I was born.

In this first yoga class, I keyed into the breath of others around me as well as my own. Feeling it and hearing it as if it were filling the nooks and crannies of my skull. Focusing on my fruit experience was like concentrating on a set of repetitions at the gym. Slow, methodical, purposeful. I began to feel a sense of intentional calmness that I had never experienced before. Weight training was a focused intensity. Very different. Both came with a feeling of strength and ultimate control, but, to my surprise, there was something about yoga that made me feel even more powerful. It's like when you have an itch on your nose and your hands are full, and you're able to will the itch away just with your mind.

After my 10-week mindfulness course at the hospital, I was thoroughly hooked on this noniron, gentle form of exercise. I was curious to explore yoga even further with newfound respect and appreciation.

I found a yoga DVD taught by a soft-spoken woman clad in ethereal, wispy white clothes. Four times per week, we practiced together in my house. She was my new workout partner. Other than walking, I was barely doing anything else physical but yoga. It kept my body moving and helped ease my mental chatter. It was during these yoga encounters that I began to discover the power of my own breath and how it could quiet the mind, which, in turn, calmed everything else. For me, the mind has always been a repository for sticky notes filled with remember to do's, ideas, memories, fears, and hopes. Those vignettes are usually flapping all over the place, but pipe in a little yoga breathing and everything starts to still.

For years, I had been using my breath in the gym to work through sets and repetitions. Knowing that the inhale happened on the easy part (such as controlling a barbell to the chest for bench press) and the exhale on the hard part (pushing the weight of the barbell off the chest), I had a high-performance technique for achieving the work. Breath gave me power. It was only through yoga that I began to discover the control over my body that my breath could provide.

Even Lamaze classes, which are all about breath, did not help me as much as the slow, rhythmic, throaty breathing that I was learning to practice through yoga. *Ujjayi* (ooh-JAH-yee) breathing, which is Sanskrit for "victorious," elongated my breath as I tried to create an audible sound against my throat. I would imagine ocean sounds, waves rolling in and onto the shore. It energized and relaxed me in ways that Lamaze never could. Control and letting go, all wrapped into one.

By my second trimester, when I was visibly pregnant, the body within my body was communicating with me. Little kicks knocked my perspective into a new place. There was a baby growing inside of me, and the job of my body was to keep it safe and nourished. Period. She kicked sense into me on a daily basis. I ate when my body told me to. I rested when I felt tired. I took deep, long breaths and walks. Over nine months, I packed 50 pounds onto my 5'4" frame. It was the ultimate experience in learning how to let go. Despite our challenges in getting pregnant, I was blessed with a relatively easy pregnancy. I do believe that being physically fit before, as well as maintaining physical activity throughout the pregnancy (right up until the day before delivery), helped me to "train" for the experience and ultimately get back on my feet afterward. When I was in labor and pushing through the pain of delivering my Butterball turkey baby (she was nine pounds, six ounces—big, just like her momma), I tried to employ Lamaze techniques, but I found myself connecting with my yoga breath instead.

When I could find stillness amid the day's chaos or my own inner chatter, I could hear a whole lot better. Yoga helped with my inner monitoring. It helped me to recognize that there were parts inside that I would *never* see. I was learning to trust.

My healthy, beautiful baby girl was finally born. Renée. To underscore her specialness, we gave her the fancy accent on her name (which she eventually dropped because it was too much work when writing!). She was named after Craig's mom who died the year before we were married. In French, Renée means "reborn."

In some ways, I viewed pregnancy as a training routine. For 40 weeks of pregnancy, I kept my eyes on the prize that would kick me in the middle of the night or make me so ravenous that I could barely wait to get my Chinese food lunch special home to eat it. (I almost swallowed the tiny staple when I tore into the fried noodles bag in the car.) It was body transformation— something I was quite comfortable with—yet netting a very different effect over time and driven by a schedule that was completely not mine to choose. With bodybuilding, I grew sharper, tighter, leaner. With pregnancy, I expanded. Both had their share of outward and inward effects.

You can do anything for the next 20 seconds.

You can do anything for the next nine months.

You can do anything.

Fitness in my thirties was the decade of beginning to learn how to let go.

To adapt.

And to recognize that no matter how hard I put my mind (and body) to something, it sometimes didn't matter.

I became less regimented because I had to. I slept when my baby slept. I skipped fitness for days at a time because I was too pooped to press on. In the first few weeks of motherhood, beyond caring for my newborn, my personal goals each day were basic, primal: taking a shower, brushing my teeth, making my bed. The simple act of straightening out my comforter and propping the pillows up was a tiny symbolic act—if I could make it, then I could *make it.* It meant I had some control over the daily chaos. It was also becoming clearer to me that control was a personal theme and that fitness through the years both helped and fed it. Through it all, I kept breathing, even though I was hyperventilating at times.

For the first seven months of Renee's life, she was exclusively breast fed. Who knew that, under my pectoralis majors, were tiny cartons of milk that were in perpetual fill mode. I kept my caloric intake up high for milk production, so the 50 pounds I had put on were not pouring off like everyone said they would. I didn't care. Watching my daughter grow and thrive on something that only I could provide was satisfying enough. I threw myself into "mommy-ing" as if I was training for a major event. I pushed through when I thought I would collapse. I ignored my fatigue when she cried in the middle of the night every two hours.

To my surprise, I did more sweating as a new mom than I did in the gym. The kind of intense perspiring from constantly juggling and schlepping, racing to beat clocks and capture firsts, tripping over plastic toys and unintended words. All-out effort coupled with lack of qualification. What a workout!

Mom's Parkinson's had progressed to a place where she could barely move or feed herself. She required around-the-clock care. I would take Renee to visit her and we'd arrive with a box of Munchkins, with a heavy emphasis on Mom's favorite, the chocolate glazed. Renee loved eating Munchkins and wearing hats, so the two of them would pass both back and forth. Mom was slow on the exchange, but Renee didn't seem to mind. The visits were playful, fun, and brief, because that's what everyone needed, so when the "How is it being a mommy?" question came up, I kept it light. This, however, meant that I didn't ask Mom about what she struggled with as a new mother. I perceived our time together as me being there for her to lean on, not the other way around.

Renee was a few months shy of two years old when Mom died. Like Dad, Mom was in her sixties when she passed on. She had been sick for so long that none of us took it as a surprise.

However, as a new mom, I felt a deeper loss than just losing my own mother. My daughter would never grow up with the influence of her grandmother. My mother would never have the joy of spoiling her granddaughter. As I grieved, layers kept unraveling. When I would fill out new patient paperwork for myself at a doctor's office, with Renee typically sitting at my side reading a book, I would feel a strange pang of reality. The family history section. If the doctor was asking, then there must be a correlation between my parents' medical history and potentially my future. I needed to do everything I could so that history would not repeat itself. *Choose healthy. Every single day.* I knew that getting more aggressive with exercise was not the answer. It would only lead to an injury I didn't have time for as a new mom. I delved deeper into yoga.

I continued to practice at home with videos, building on the foundational elements I had established during pregnancy. Practice, in general, is the ongoing commitment to just keep working at something. Yoga practice was my true pivotal shift toward learning how to connect with the power of the mind. The body, as I was witnessing more and more while taking care of another body but my own, was always in flux. The mind could be constant as the sun. I found that, while I was engaged in the methodical asanas and the breathing for 30–40 minutes, I couldn't really think much. This calmness would spill over into my day even after I got off the mat. Yoga had a profound impact on my mental state.

One day, I discovered that there was yoga being taught at our gym. It was free with membership. Every week, I would head out after dinner to catch the evening class. The teacher was a cross between Zen master and rocker dude. Buddha meets badass. I could relate. I liked the methodical consistency of working the exact same sequence of poses, week after week. This predictability made it easier for me to follow along and recognize my progress. The poses were challenging, and I could barely do many of them. I liked this.

Yoga tapped me on the shoulder and said, "Hey, don't underestimate me—I can kick your butt, too." This particular type of yoga pointed out that my hip flexibility wasn't there. It showed me that my balance was off. It shifted my bodybuilding mindset about muscle symmetry for aesthetics to symmetry for wholeness. If you do one part, you need to address the other. A yin-yang. It made it evident that my body would not cooperate just because I wanted it to. I could feel myself drawing from the inner strength I had built up in my twenties. Unbeknownst to me, I was practicing Ashtanga yoga, one of the most physical yoga styles there is. Ashtanga yoga literally means "eight-limbed yoga" in Sanskrit. These "limbs" work in concert as they focus on various parts of a total being, from posture to strength to bliss. I practiced the Primary Series in this six-part series for about two years, never having advanced beyond the first series. I barely grazed the surface. It was humbling.

Ashtanga yoga also furthered my physical strength and flexibility, which I had lost a lot of during pregnancy. The movements were methodical, repetitive, rhythmic, predictable, and boring, but in a helpful, meditative way. While on the mat, I would envision that I'm in a little boat that seats one, bobbing in the water, everything around me, nothing around me, with two oars that I keep moving in and out of the water. I can't tell if I'm heading east or west, north or south, but I feel that I am moving. This practice helped me develop willpower, mind-body awareness, and confidence in my ability to get my footing as a new mom, and also as me.

Practicing yoga taught me how to breathe actively. When sitting for a blood test, mammogram, or some other medical procedure that made me anxious, I would start breathing like I was hyperventilating, only its effect was quite the opposite. This long, even *Ujjayi* breathing was building my internal fire in ways I never got from weight training.

Having success in powerlifting and bodybuilding bolstered my ego when I needed it, and yoga humbled me back down in size when I was ready for it. I was not the strongest, the most flexible, or the best in any yoga class—and that was OK. People would plop down into *Hanumanasana* (monkey pose, which is a flat-out split) like they were gliding into a warm tub. This was impossible for my body. I'd attempt a headstand by a wall to steady myself only to be thumping out of the pose every few seconds. From my early days as a ballerina to my recent years in the gym, I was always surrounded by mirrors. The mirrors helped to validate my external progress. There were no mirrors in the yoga studios. With yoga, my reflection was only in my mind's eye. Rather than just seeing the literal image of myself, I was drawing from mental images tied to experiences, memories, relationships, people, and places. The first time I heard my daughter laugh. Her baby smell. Craig's voice. Dad's hand when he'd hold mine and walk me to school. Mom's smile the first day she saw Renee. The smell of childhood jelly shoes at the sprinklers during summer. Being one with my fruit. Yoga slowly taught me that my intentional letting go could be equally as powerful as my death grip on things.

After spending an hour on the mat a few times each week for a few years, I felt calmer, more grounded, more peaceful. Good qualities for a new mommy. My pregnancy weight was slowly coming off. My energy level was returning.

I was coming back to me. Or so I thought.

This version of me was not exactly where I left off a few years prior.

Something was different.

I felt so peaceful, yet so terribly restless.

I was approaching 40. Forty? Wasn't my mother just 40 and waiting for me after school, looking like the most glamorous mother in the world? I grew up with the influence of a glam mom who was always in high heels and a long coat with a fur collar. With perfect, pink, smiling lips. My daughter had the mom in leggings, sports bra, sweaty ponytail, and no makeup.

Did Renee think I was glamorous?

What mattered most to me was that she saw me as strong.

But did *I* think I was strong?

I felt so peaceful, yet so terribly restless.

GOING BACK (IN BLACK)

Ten years of practicing yoga had made it officially stick for me in my day-to-day routine, particularly in thought and in breath. The dialogue in my head had begun to evolve toward calming me down when life got crazy, instead of fueling the frenzy. *Honor the chaos in your head. Welcome it into the room, and then escort it out the door.* This statement helped me to meditate on not fighting to push out the thoughts of deadlines, schedules, to-do lists, and what if's pinging against the walls of my skull. Instead, I imagined a calm, soft-spoken adult, someone very much like my mom, lovingly putting her arm around a panicked thought. I could see her leaning into it to whisper, "It's OK," and then gently guiding the negative thought to the door.

I went to a great yoga studio each week where the people became like family. Comprised of men and women of all ages, sizes, abilities, and goals, they were the most forgiving, kind, nonjudgmental people I had ever met. It's true what they say about yogis! I picked up a phrase along the way from the group: *Focus on your own mat.* It would come in handy when my inner competitor would try to catch an envious glimpse of the perfectly stacked knees of the girl half my age doing cow face pose (*Gomukhasana*). I would practice breath work (*pranayama*) in traffic or right before bed to ground my thoughts and relax my body.

Still, I felt restless. Now, at the milestone age of 40, a part of me was longing to go back in time. Maybe I could find some part of the younger me if I picked up my old intensity at the gym. I had to see. I craved the physical *grr* that only hard training had provided. Other than a foray into marathoning, Craig had remained consistent with his powerlifting all these years, so I knew he'd be there to spot me if I needed him to.

Could I go back to competing like I did in my twenties? Did I *want* to go back to competing? Would I body build again? Or powerlift? Could my body sustain either of those sports anymore? I felt different. I looked different. In my old fitness mindset, I had merely taken a little time off from weight training to heal from overtraining. This was typically a week or two or maybe a month, not

10 years! Even though I never stopped working out in the gym, I felt like I had been in a beast-mode coma. Now, I was coming back around, but while my mind was eager to get back to where I left off, my body was floundering. Ten years older, parts positioned a bit differently in certain places. Never mind would I or could I body build again— *should* I? The training part, sure. I was excited for the hard work and the personal test. The competing in a bikini on a stage part in the "master's division"? No way! I didn't even wear a bikini on the beach (I'd wear the top, but only with a skirted bottom). But if I wasn't training for competition, what was I training for?

I had finally settled into my role as a mom. I wasn't sweating all the time and juggling baby paraphernalia like car seats and diaper bags. With my daughter in school all day and then in after-school activities, I gained back significant chunks of time in my day to devote to full-time freelance writing. My head was clear enough to take a hard look at my fitness. But without a set goal waiting for me at the top of a hill, it was unclear what my exercise focus should look like. I just knew I needed a focus.

I went for smaller personal goals. Getting back to the main lifts again, like bench pressing or deadlifting. Or increasing a bench press by a few pounds or reps. Breaking the 10-minute-per-mile barrier when running on the treadmill. Getting into more challenging yoga poses, particularly arm balances like firefly (*Titibasana*). Arm balances were my yogi-meets-HercuLisa moments because, while they helped me work my patience and balance, they also tapped into my upper body strength.

I'd go to the gym 3–4 times per week, usually in the early mornings, and do an hour workout that included cardio and weight training. I dabbled in my old moves, combining the best of powerlifting with bodybuilding. Like heavy squats followed by five sets of high-rep, low-weight leg extensions and, on another day, heavy benching with cable crossovers and dumbbell flies, and always some kind of cardio to get that therapeutic sweat I loved. Sometimes I'd train in the evening with Craig, and Renee would come with us to hang out in the childcare playroom. Training with Craig brought me back into the fold of working out with the guys again.

I could rest on my fitness laurels, start sentences with "I used to…," and still feel relevant, competitive, worthy. But if I didn't quickly pick up where HercuLisa had left off, I would run the risk of losing all that I spent years building up. A physique, a number on a bench press, a reputation, a persona, an identity. HercuLisa's existence was synonymous with the gym. If I let this all go, if I just did yoga from this point forward, would that be enough? Would I become the nimble old lady without HercuLisa grit? I felt compelled to hang onto the grit until my fingers couldn't grip anymore.

I started bench pressing again. A lot. And heavy. I had inched back up to 135 pounds on the bar for a few reps. I even paused one of these reps, which basically means I let the bar rest on my chest before I pressed it up into the air. Just like the old days! Without the momentum of springing the weight off my chest, the lift was that much more difficult and impressive. *You still got it! Maybe you could do a bench press meet again?* The ego's rant compelled me to add a five-pound plate to each side of the bar. To feed my ego, I also started doing pull-ups again. In my heyday, I could do 10 of those babies in a row. In my forties, I could still hoist myself up six or seven times. Nothing beat the feeling of being so strong in a way that women typically were not. Women have less upper body strength, blah, blah.

But lifting like the old days came at a price. I was getting tweaked and torn. I'd wake up with a stiff neck or a pinched deltoid, which would make it impossible to function that day. Out of nowhere, I developed a bad case of tendonitis in my left bicep. One morning, I woke up with stiffness in my left shoulder. Aches and pains had been my body's way of talking to me and I liked feeling sore. It made me feel accomplished. A stiff left shoulder would typically last a day or two, and I'd move on. This time, the pain persisted for days, weeks, months. I had to baby myself all over again, including no heavy bench pressing or yoga inversions. Handstands and headstands hurt like heck. Even downward dog was killing me. It took a year-long case of bicep tendonitis, along with lots of physical therapy, to finally reach the revelation that I couldn't go back. My mind wanted to fight it, but my body didn't agree.

Try going forward.

A quiet little voice, and I'm not even sure it was mine, reset my point of view.

My love of fitness started with giving a pair of gold dumbbells a chance, with running for the first time down Kissena Boulevard, with bopping along to an exercise tape when all I ever used the TV for was after-school vegetation. Up until now, I hadn't considered the value of any of the current fitness trends. I had been set in my old ways, but, out of frustration, I was ready to give anything a try. Craig and I caught an informercial for a workout program. It was a series of DVDs with a host of insane workouts packed in. The program suggested a six-times-per-week workout over 12 weeks with each workout anywhere from 40 to 60 minutes long. Sign us up! Who better to attack this program with me than my old workout partner? Neither of us would say, "Let's skip today," so, just like in the old days, we both trained hard and pushed each other. This DVD series gave me everything I needed at the time: intensity, focus, a challenge, a routine, a finite goal to train for, plus the flexibility to do it whenever I could squeeze it in. I took it on vacation. I did it early in the morning before the day began or in the evening with Craig while Renee watched her crazy parents jump around for an hour.

For the first time ever, my workouts were sans equipment. Granted, yoga only required a mat, but I never thought of yoga as working out. It was a practice. But now, exercising in a way that was just simply me against me was an exciting challenge. No weights, no machines, no newfangled bands or ropes to create resistance. I was the resistance. Every single movement was about jumping, running in place, push-ups, balance, moving as quickly as I could for 30-second bouts. I loved it! I had discovered a new way to stay gritty.

"Me against me" may have been the killer mindset that propelled me through the hour-long workouts, but it was the purity of the workouts—the ability to do them anywhere, anytime, in any way that suited my needs at that very moment—that made me unite with the simplicity of self. I could improvise the movements if I didn't have the DVD playing in front of me, like if we were on vacation and couldn't get to a gym. I could work out right there in the hotel room. I could push hard or pull back without any measurements of pounds or tracking repetitions. All I needed was me, short bouts of intensity, and a stopwatch. This opened my mind to seeing fitness in ways that I hadn't considered *ever*. There was something so pure and simple about being able to do what I called a "prison cell workout," which was basically exercise in the smallest space with no equipment—nothing other than yourself.

My regimented thoughts about what a workout had to look like were being challenged at the perfect time. I started looking at the gym schedules for group fitness classes. There were all kinds of new trends going on that I had not been paying attention to: TRX classes, boot camps, kickboxing, Zumba, and CrossFit, just to name a few. I allowed myself the opportunity to dabble in new things and, as I continually surprised my muscles with unfamiliar activity, I found my mind opening up, too. *Give it a try. Let yourself be vulnerable. Be comfortable with uncomfortable.* The internal mantras were coming back to me, but with a different spin and spirit.

I had always trained with competitive male athletes, but here I was in exercise rooms surrounded by estrogen. The same women greeted me each week as we all faced the mirror. No one pointing fingers, no whispering behind my back. This was a community of women of all ages, all fitness levels, who just wanted to exercise in a friendly, encouraging environment. The instructors all had their unique styles and personalities, and I was beginning to appreciate the teachings and motivation they generously imparted to their students.

My little girl with the wacky parents who were always training, arm wrestling, doing push-ups, and reading food labels made me ponder my legacy. The dumbbells Dad had passed on to me were my cue to start something he was so passionate about yet couldn't achieve. What would the inscription on my torch to Renee say?

Craig and I had fitness standards that we set high for ourselves, so naturally they were high for our daughter, too. However, Renee was independent and introspective, and from a super-young age she knew what she did and didn't like. Dressing up, coloring, doing puzzles, watching her favorite movies such as *The Wizard of Oz* were among her top choices. And reading. Oh, how she loved to read. Many of her favorite activities circled around sitting quietly. Sometimes I swear she would look at Craig and me working out in the basement, a book in her lap, as if to say, "What is wrong with you guys?" The neighbors had two girls, both around Renee's age; they were natural athletes, always sprinting all over our adjoining lawns, climbing trees like monkeys, and kicking soccer balls with impressive power. Our little cutie, analytical and calm from the start, would watch them bouncing around like flies against a window.

We exposed Renee to every sport imaginable—dance, soccer, basketball, tennis, gymnastics, swimming, running—hoping she would find her fitness passion. Even with Craig coaching her soccer and basketball teams, she didn't like either one all that much. Too much running made her side hurt. Too much sweating made her feel too hot. The other kids on the teams were pushing and shoving. It just wasn't her style.

Dance was Renee's passion for quite a few years. She started with a combo class—jazz, tap, and ballet, and she loved it. We did what any overly zealous parent does these days when their kid shows an inkling of an interest in something: we double the exposure! More is better. More is what everyone else is doing, so there's this inordinate pressure to keep up. There's no middle ground for kids and sports in our neck of the woods. Travel teams, private coaching, strength training sessions, double sessions, longer classes, more of everything. If we didn't accelerate the classes, then she'd be at risk of falling behind, which would lead to her becoming the kid who didn't make a team or get a prime position in a dance formation, which would ultimately lead to underachiever placement in every category of life!

Renee really enjoyed dance for a while. We could see it in her smile each time we'd pick her up from one of her classes. She liked the music, which ranged from soft and classical in her ballet class to Broadway hits in lyrical class to pop in hip-hop. She loved the frilly costumes, enjoyed her friends, and was a part of something that appeared to make her feel good about herself. Plus, she was being physically active almost every day. As fitness-focused parents, what more could we ask?

By age seven, she had been asked to join the dance troupe, which seemed like she had hit the lottery. This came with a rigorous schedule of four dance classes per week. On top of that were the troupe practices, many of which gobbled up entire Sundays. More recitals, more numbers to perfect, more expensive costumes to purchase. As long as she loved it, we were happy to support her efforts. The more often she danced, the more I was brought back to my old dance experiences. As she would come out of her 7–8 pm class, I'd see a bunch of women sauntering into the 8–9 pm adult hip-hop class. *Hmm.* I hadn't taken a dance class in over 35 years. Could this be fun, or would it give me PTSD? I needed to find out.

The owner of the studio, who was probably 50 at the time, was also the hip-hop teacher. Dressed in black leggings, a cool tie-dye tank top, and black sneakers, she looked nothing like Ms.

Hauser. I walked into the room, the room where I had seen my daughter dance for years, and I felt triggered. It all rushed back in—the wall-to-wall mirrors, the scuffed hardwood floor, the ballet bar against the wall that I would death grip to transfer the tension inside of me, the formation of girls standing around and waiting for class to begin. I remembered my breath and took another look at the mirror's reflection. The little girl in the unforgiving baby pink leotard was all grown up now. One hip-hop class in, and I was hooked. Maybe it was the music (remixes of old stuff and the new stuff my daughter was listening to), the moves (all attitude combinations, and a ton of athletic stuff like jumps and worms), and the way it made me feel. Fun, free, tough, young.

I was thrilled to have one rigorous, fun hour each week to complement my fitness at the gym. I had found myself a new kind of fitness. In true goal-oriented fashion, I was suddenly signed up for the recitals. Two, in fact. One group number included jumping off folding chairs to "Push It" by Salt-n-Pepa, while the other had tombstones and black sweatshirts with bones and a skull over the hood, which completely zipped up over the head. It was hard to see and breathe. The music was "Boom Boom Pow" by the Black Eyed Peas. The last time I had performed on stage was a bodybuilding show more than 15 years ago. This time, the other people on the stage were counting on each other, not competing against each other. Renee thought it was the coolest thing that I was in the recital, too. Finally, there was something fitness-related that we were both connected by!

But that didn't last very long. As she entered her preteen years and the Pattys from my childhood began to show up for her, her dance passion fizzled. There was drama. There was burnout. There was self-doubt. It reminded me how hard it can be for all of us to find our personal fitness groove. In many ways, it was way harder for her than me because there was a clear expectation from her generation to partake in some kind of physical, sport-related activity from a young age. Everyone did. Plus, she had obsessive parents. All we wanted was for her to love fitness like we did, so it could be a healthy habit for life. Just move your body.

As a family, we played tennis, went on long hikes, worked out in the basement, jumped rope, and shot hoops at the Y. During a run with gymnastics, Renee told us she wanted to stop. "I don't like these things," she said as she pointed to the tiniest callouses forming on her hands. Craig and I laughed because "those things" were the crusty battle scars we loved. When we'd do our arm wrestles after dinner (eventually, she decided to join this family antic), I'd look her square in the eye right before we'd begin and say, "Where does strength come from?" It became our little mantra and, every time I'd ask, she'd recite the answer, "From within."

But here again was Craig's and my inability to just chill out. On days when Renee would pop down to the basement while we'd be exercising, she'd leave minutes later because we went all Marine drill sergeant on her. *Try this! Do this!* We had to learn how and when to pull back. I had to act like none of it mattered that much. (Like when kids potty train—if you push too hard, they show you who *really* is in charge.) All this was easier said than done.

Renee was growing up, and I was still working on that letting go thing. I couldn't control the things she gravitated toward. She was going to find her own path no matter what exposure we gave her. In middle school she played softball and field hockey. In high school she played on the varsity tennis team. It was such a thrill to cheer her on, even though Craig and I were instructed to not overdo it with the screaming. Screaming parents were a magnet for the thing she disliked most: the spotlight. She was more of an athlete than I ever was at her age, and with hand-eye coordination that made her jock daddy proud. Eventually, Renee signed up for a membership at our gym and everything started to shift for her.

All those years of fitness exposure, although unwelcome at times, were a part of Renee's upbringing. We constantly modeled behavior that we believed in for ourselves, for our family. Our message was consistent as well as our actions. It's one thing to have one parent like this, but two? Renee handled us very well. Once she began to explore her own experiences at the gym, and she was about 16 years old at this point, we could see her interest in fitness blossoming.

Craig and I wanted to give Renee the tools to always feel confident in the gym, so we taught her how to use the machines, gave her tips on which exercises hit which body parts, and explained the tenets of designing her own fitness routine. Cardio, strength, flexibility, speed, balance—we educated her on these things. Gym knowledge leads to power. We challenged her to think about her personal goals, goals of any kind, so that she could take the steps toward reaching them.

Throughout her high school years and then beyond, Renee and I tested out many different forms of fitness together. This became our new way of enjoying mom-daughter time together. We quickly got hooked on spin classes, 5K races, hardcore boxing classes (taught by a former Marine), SUP (standup paddle) yoga on the ocean, barre classes (and woke up sore the next day in places where we didn't even know we had muscle), and intense cardio classes where we flipped oversized truck tires for fun. We hiked the "Lemon Squeeze" trail in New Paltz, New York. There's a sick part at the end of the hike where you actually climb up a ladder between two boulder crevices to "squeeze" yourself to the summit. Through all this experimentation, I had found myself aligned with the best female workout partner of my life. One of the most amazing parts of working out together was witnessing her personal power development.

By now, the entire Safran family was hooked on fitness. Plus, I had a new fitness groove that was based on being flexible enough to dabble in unchartered workout territory. I could be more open-minded around fitness. I was 50 years old and making progress with this work in progress.

BEYOND A DUMBBELL

The numbers are in.

I've been influenced by fitness all 50 years of my life.

I've been actively engaged in fitness for almost 70 percent of my life.

I've lifted millions of pounds.

Counted enough repetitions to also equal the millions.

Spent well over 10,000 hours in a gym, the sweet spot for honing a skill to perfection, according to Malcolm Gladwell's book, *Outliers*.

Competed in more than a dozen bodybuilding and powerlifting competitions.

Ran more than fifteen 5K and 10K foot races.

Wore through over 100 pairs of sneakers, including my first pair of beloved Puma Clydes.

Participated in countless fitness trends, including 1980s' aerobics tapes, kickboxing classes, candle-lit spin classes, tire-flipping classes, TRX classes, and super-intense classes designed to keep the heart rate in an optimal zone, just to name a few.

I started this fitness journey with minimal awareness of my body to possessing full control over it, then lost control only to redefine it, all over the last five decades.

When I get on the treadmill these days, I stare at the buttons in front of me and I literally watch time tick away. The seconds go by so fast, yet the distance can feel like an eternity, especially if I'm scheduled to run a few miles or I'm just flat-out not in the mood that day. While time rolls forward on a conveyor belt, I contemplate it.

When the run starts, I might be inner-chanting: *You can't do this. You'll never maintain that pace.* Yeah, I still have the "good and evil" dialogue playing out at times.

But when my favorite song comes on Spotify (these days it's "Cold as Ice" by Foreigner), I lose myself in the beat, keeping up with the lyrics as I mentally sing along or sometimes mouth along, but I'm sure I look insane doing that. I celebrate time when I only have two minutes left before a run is complete and my thoughts shift to encouragement. *Hang in there. You got this.*

The start button triggers "go," and I do. The pause button is ideal for an unexpected need to pee or a shoelace undone. The cooldown I rarely hit because it never provides the pace or time that I need at that precise moment, so I just lower the controls manually. (Emphasis on *controls*!) It's the red stop button, the one that looks like an emergency abort, that gives me the most angst. Sometimes I accidentally hit it with my hand and then I need to start all over again. If I purposely hit stop, I wonder if I will be able to start again precisely where I left off.

Fitness is not an elixir, but it is a trickster. It makes me think I'm better than I am when I'm really just your average Joe. It pumps me up when I feel like I've got nothing, and suddenly I've got something. It distracts me when I struggle or get scared. It helps me work through the yucky feelings left over after saying or doing dumb stuff. It just makes me feel good. I still experience a twinge of guilt when I skip a workout or eat like it's the day after a bodybuilding show. I keep working on letting go of things that don't matter that much in the grand scheme. But the grand scheme is the final act, and very little will matter at that moment, so, the heck with it—if I can't let go, then I'll just let go of letting go.

I also try hard to let go of what *does* matter because the tightness of my grip changes nothing. It just makes my hands hurt. With each year that passes, I think about some of my go-to mantras as well as some new ones. These little phrases help me to coach me. They assist in setting a positive point of view. When I actively frame my thoughts, my thoughts can better guide my actions.

You can.

You will.

Just do your best.

Just let it go.

Like fitness, life is hard work. Some days you just want to skip it. Other days you wonder what's the point. But most days, you realize it's what you're built to do because it's what you're built from. Fitness requires consistency, discipline, dedication, and a commitment to not give up on yourself even when everything in your being is telling you to do so. Honing those skills through fitness allows you to call on them and pull them through in other aspects of daily life.

At the same time, fitness is as easy as blowing the delicate fuzz off a dandelion. All it takes is one big exhale—or one step forward, one dumbbell curled, one head bowed at the end of yoga class with a final *Namaste*.

I had this beautiful red angora sweater in high school. It was my first expensive sweater, a special gift from my parents. I treasured it. It was so fuzzy, soft, and fragile. When I'd run my hands up and down my arms to bask in the luxuriousness, the little hairs from the knit stood up with electricity. It literally made me feel alive! When I wasn't wearing it, I kept the sweater folded up in a plastic bag, gently tucked inside a drawer. And when my friend got mad at me for not loaning it to her for the weekend (she was infamous for destroying her own clothes), I had to deal with her wrath and my own guilt. I'm learning to treat my body like my angora sweater—like I will never own something this special ever again in my lifetime. A gift that comes with the responsibility to take good care of it.

As I look over my shoulder at where I've been, I see my fitness trail. One long, sometimes bumpy, never straight, pretty much continuous line that has kept me on my course to physical and mental connectivity. Fitness has helped me figure things out; it has taught me to strive toward letting go not only when I have to but also when I choose to; and it has given me strength inside and outside of the gym.

I was in the slow cooker for the months leading up to a competition, to inside a bubble the day of competition, to feeling like I'm in a time capsule today. *In.* The perfect word to describe where fitness has taken me all these years. Such a tiny word. It's ironic that I spent so many years working on my physical self—my muscles and fast-twitch fibers, stamina, and flexibility. Places I could see, things that could be tested and measured, but it's the immeasurable inner strength that fitness has brought me that makes me feel alive. If it weren't for those darn mirrors at the gym, I could easily be tricked into thinking that I am still 25 years old, getting ready to train with the guys, preparing for some competition four months out.

As I do what I can to "ease" into this fifth decade of life, I witness my body and mind dueling in ways they never did before. They used to work together much more harmoniously. When I decide that running outside on a beautiful day is exactly what I need, I'm later reminded by my aching knee joints that running on the hard concrete was a bad idea. Maybe it's the sneakers and the soles that are too worn down. Nah, it's me. When my yoga teacher says to join her in hero pose (*Virasana*), I realize the only heroes here are my kneecaps for not exploding from sitting in a position that is meant for toddlers. Mind gets me into trouble by painting a beautiful picture of the infinite things Body can do if I put Mind to it. Mind is a troublemaker!

Who I used to be is forever carved into my heartstrings. It's my hamstrings that are starting to give me trouble. My muscles are tight because I'm not doing yoga as regularly as I used to. My knees hurt if I run too many times in one week. I have low back pain if I sit at my desk too long. This creakiness is new for my body, or maybe I'm just less tolerant. Sometimes I wonder what would happen if I hopped off the fitness trail. Would I completely fall to pieces? Enter inertia? Or would I feel free?

These days, I keep my locker combination hidden in my iPhone so that, when it's time to get my coat and bag, I don't stare at the shiny, metal object and secretly say, "What's the combination again?" I had my old combination memorized like a song, but then I lost the lock a few years ago and had to start over with all new numbers and a new color (now silver, formerly purple). I keep jumbling up which color had which combination. Plus, I can barely see the numbers without my reading glasses, but those are *in* the locker. The only other time I had this memory lapse at the gym was when I was pregnant. I spent fifteen minutes jiggering the lock. Just as the front desk guy was about to clip it, I realized that I had been yanking on the wrong lock. Now, at 50, I can only chalk this kind of experience up to my short-term memory being a vindictive sloth that would rather mess with me than remember three stinking numbers.

I used to count to sets of 50 when bodybuilding. Now it's a number that equals an accumulation of self—a compiling of every set, rep, drop of sweat, and head game that I have invested in over most of my life. It's a commitment notch on the lifting belt to myself that I made a long time ago to exercise. To make it as mandatory as breath itself. My motives were singular and, yes, superficial, at the time—a bigger this, a more refined that, a win, a personal best, a toned physique—but the cumulative effect continues to blossom in ways I never set out for. As with anything you commit to, you just have to hold on long enough to get over the discomfort of the hump. Humps are designed to slow us down. If we don't muster up the drive to accelerate over them, they will get in the way.

There's a secret formula for making fitness a part of your normal life.

Here it is: *Take one step.*

Just one.

Simple, right?

There are no excuses (*I ate so much junk this weekend, so why bother*), rationalizations (*I'm not much of an exercise person*), barters (*If I don't work out today, I'll do it tomorrow*) or pity (*I can't even run a block*). The trick to navigating a hump is acknowledging it, bowing to it with respect, surrendering to the uncomfortable feeling that it seems like Mount Everest, and then simply pressing on anyway. *Just one step.*

These days, when I feel the iron in my hands, I instantly connect with HercuLisa. The iron always starts off feeling cold when I first pick it up; my body heat transfers to it in seconds. I absorb it; it absorbs me.

But as wonderful as it is to be the *ma'am* who puts on old sweats (I still have my favorite light gray, frayed-at-the-sleeves sweatshirt from 33 years ago) and doesn't (well, almost doesn't) bother to look in the mirror before she heads out the door, it's all a trick. Because I am half a century old and, while my inner badass is spry and spunky, and I still train as beastly as I can (but not every time), I'm getting older. I'm the oldest I've ever been!

I'm discovering that this is the portion of the program when I need to be even more mindful about fitness. It's no longer about just doing what I've always done, or simply what I feel like, but being smarter. Now I'm finding that 6–8 sets, not 10–12, are more than enough. Sometimes even four will suffice. My goals are different. I am not looking to get bigger, stronger, and more refined for competition. I just want to stay healthy and fit while still being able to get out of bed in the morning without too much cracking and groaning. I want to be able to hike the "Lemon Squeeze" with Renee like we've done every year for the last five years on our mother-daughter excursions. I want energy to maximize each day I'm fortunate enough to have. I want to be Craig's workout partner for many more decades, and my goal is to let him lean on me for a spot just as often as I do him.

However, I know that, at some point, there's going to be a version of me unable to keep up with the old me that will forever live inside. When will this happen? Who knows and who cares. Therefore, I keep going. Keep breathing. Just one step. Over and over again.

I recently trained for my very first half-marathon. It was empowering to set a fresh, new goal and to take the slow, methodical, hard-working steps toward achieving it. With all my old neck tweaks, I never thought my body could sustain the impact of excessive pounding on pavement. But I wanted to try! I started off real slow with the training. I also mixed up running outside with running on a lower-impact treadmill. I skipped runs if my body was too sore. I walked sometimes when my lungs burned too hard to maintain my pace up a hill. I also pushed myself to go faster or farther, just not every time. A slow-and-steady-finishes-the-race approach allowed me to victoriously cross the finish line. Bigger than the race itself was the personal test. Just as committed to the consistent training, I was equally committed to stopping if my body couldn't take it. This is not quitting; it's strategic training.

Keeping iron in my diet is still on the top of my fitness list. Weight-bearing exercises are proven to keep the bones strong, so I make sure to lift a few times a week. Each trip to the gym is like a visit to an all-you-can-eat buffet: I load up my plate with a variety of things (a few curls here, a few pulls there, some cardio, some stretching, jump rope, etc.), but the difference these days is knowing that I don't have to go back for a second serving. More is not better. More can be gluttony. More can equal injury. More is no more.

In this fifth decade of life I'm surprisingly open to trying new things at the gym and setting different goals. I give much of the credit to my daughter who pushed me out of my "comfort zone" with spin classes and group fitness classes. I was a workout loner for a while. (I can still be some days.) Training with others who span the ages of 20-something to 60-something reminds me that there's a shared energy in a room that we all feed off of and contribute to. The instructors are knowledgeable and supportive. They inspire and push me, and many of them are way less than half my age. I love learning from them.

For the longest time, I've wanted to be able to do a jump rope crossover. It falls in the category of "parlor tricks"—those things that are just fun and cool to do. I've been wanting to do this since I first watched Rocky Balboa whipping the rope around while training for a big fight. I looked up videos on YouTube to understand how to break down the technique. I practiced at the gym, purposely in public, where others could witness my blunders. No use of mirrors—just going by feel. Practice, practice, practice My ego was on the backburner as I approached this new learning as a student and not someone who could just "pick up a weight" and grunt through. I'm proud to say that, after many months of working at it, I have achieved the crossover. Not even close to mastered it but enough to make me proud of myself for sticking with the goal. For sticking with the fumbles. For honoring that I'm not good at it and so what. I trip a lot and get rope welts across my arms and butt, but when I do achieve a few loops, I feel like screaming, "Adrian!"

I've heard that sitting at a desk all day is the new smoking, so I do my best to get up off my duff every hour. A wearable is just what I need to keep me on point with my steps these days. The little silhouette girl that pops up on my wrist gets so excited to take a few steps with me. I can't let her down.

I recently bought a new pair of Puma Clydes. I was in Macy's with my sister, who does a great job reminding me of stories from our past. (She has the gift of remembering everything.) It was no surprise then that, when I saw the Clydes on the shelf, I was instantly drawn to them. It's been close to 40 years since I had a pair. Seems they're hot again, and since the category of fashion sneakers is acceptable for a "girl" my age, I got myself a pair in black-and-white suede. Back when I was 12, they made me feel cool and energized, ready to take on my day. Funny how some things never change.

At every gym we've ever joined there has always been one older couple working out. They always wore workout attire that was popular 10 years prior, and they constantly sipped on protein shakes. Craig and I were always sure they were in their fifties or sixties. Old! Craig and I are now that couple. The remarkable comes from my long-time workout partner still being very involved in training and powerlifting competition. This continues to inspire me. Craig recently went to Sweden to lift in the IPF (International Powerlifting Federation) World Championship. This was a goal of his for 30 years! He snagged the bronze medal for his weight class. He traveled across the globe to compete in the Masters' Class (age 50+) and won! Craig epitomizes a certain Dorian Gray, gym-style, that still inspires me to follow suit.

I'm no fitness superstar. Sure, I had my 15 minutes of fame a couple of times, but, these days, I'm really pretty average. I have cellulite just like everyone else and skin you can pinch. I eat crap. (OK, not really that often.) I do embarrassing things like flying off the treadmill because I tripped. (Yes, this happened.) I'm still young enough (on the inside) to care that I looked like an idiot, and still too proud to say, "Someone please help me up." But evolved enough to laugh at myself. My friends exercise, their spouses exercise, and so do their kids. Thankfully, this next generation of adults is deeply invested in personal fitness. This moving your body thing is not a novel idea these days. We all know what we're *supposed* to do.

Fitness taught me so much about my body—how to connect with it, understand it, make it work hard for me, listen to it, cherish it, not be so hard on it (physically and emotionally), push it, laugh at it, and respect it for all the amazing things it has done and still can do. It's the aggregate of exercise over the last few decades—not one thing or experience—that has created the biggest impact in my life. I've made it a habit that's as necessary as breathing. I've also created muscle memory, which is a real scientific by-product of consistent exercise over time. The muscles remember how to work and how to function. I wonder, though, if my mental memory fails over time, will my muscle memory still be able to recall?

Recently, Renee and I tried ziplining. There I was, high up in the trees somewhere in Pennsylvania, tethered to a wire that would lead me from one obstacle to the next. Some parts were pretty easy, and if I was able to let go of my fear and just leap forward, I made it to the next platform. (Barely sometimes!) Other obstacles had swinging ropes and poles to test my upper body strength. I had to dig deep, hold on tight, and move ahead with warrior fierceness. *You can do this.* I heard myself saying this as I went flying through the sky. Of course, I had never done *this* before. The goal was simply getting to the other side. The feeling was pure adrenaline. Those things were way familiar to me. Maybe that's my true muscle memory. Always remembering how good it feels to feel strong.

As I enter into my fifties, I am seeing signs of strange things to come. My sweats used to be the pants I wore. Now I'm sweating when I'm not even doing anything aerobic (menopause is so much fun); my body aches in odd places like the pinky toe I broke in the gym 25 years ago when a weight dropped on it; and I get a kick out of younger people who politely ask me about the 40-pound dumbbell near my feet— "Ma'am, are you using that?"—and look at me like that would be impossible. (By the way, it's not!)

Reflecting on my journey with fitness I can better see the big picture, despite not having my glasses from Costco at easy reach. Why did I start fitness back in my teens? It was to cope with my insecurities and frustrations, to help me navigate the difficult teenage years, and to escape my fear of repeating Dad's struggles. I started engaging in fitness To Control Me.

Once I had a handle on how much power I had over me, fitness continued to be my main outlet for discovery. I did it to feel good and to look good. It was how I strengthened a healthy relationship with my husband. It was the constant testing of self. *How far could I push? What more could I do? What could I prove to myself? To others?* I continued my fitness To Define Me. By around age 40, after over 20 years of consistent daily exercise, my fitness was necessary To Be Me. It became like breathing.

After years and years of this lifestyle commitment, and as I continue to grow more comfortable in my own skin, fitness is still what I do for the reasons stated. But there's another layer now that didn't exist before: To Extend Me. My goal is to be around for the long haul, and to be as healthy and strong as possible. If I can keep my bones strong, my muscle mass high, and my heart healthy, then I'm doing my part. Guess that puts me full circle to wanting To Control Me. But at 50, I understand that that is an impossible goal. (Hey, you can't fault me for trying!)

More than just striving for good health, I do hope that fitness allows me opportunities To Evolve Me. Working through the body is a conduit to the spirit. My goal is to figure out how to work my body, or not, to bring me closer to who I am and why I'm here.

Fitness also provides a direct route to my mind. And it is there where I continue to find strength. I've trained it, or maybe it has trained me, to think a certain way or remember a specific movement. There are days when I walk into the gym and I don't even think about what to do—my body just takes over. A different kind of muscle memory.

When I was as young as kindergarten age, adults used to say that I was an old soul. I never thought much of it until I started working out. Through exercise, I began to connect with an inner strength that I didn't quite know I had. Especially evident to me when I began to train for competitive powerlifting and bodybuilding, this strength allowed me to push through with my mind when my body was tapping out. But where did this come from? The strength was really all in my head, or so I thought.

There was a huge bodybuilder dude at one of our gyms years ago who kept to himself even more than the other bodybuilders. Very quiet and super-focused. He lifted like a beast and was built like a house. We did the obligatory head nod whenever we saw each other, but other than that, few words were exchanged. One day, he struck up a conversation with Craig. They were talking about training philosophies when he said, "There's one person here who has more heart than anyone I've ever seen." Craig ran through the list of suspects, but this guy kept nodding no. Finally, he said, "It's someone you know pretty well." He was pointing at me. "She has more heart than anyone around here." *Me, heart?* Well, I *had* a heart. I was compassionate and caring, always the first one to ask, "How are you?" and stick around for the answer.

Heart—the thumping, beating engine that I train every single day. I work it hard some days, raising it to max levels when I run hills on the tread. I work it gently when I take a slow stroll with my workout partner after work. I train it moderately when I try to hold an inversion pose (headstand) for two minutes straight or carry laundry up and down the stairs in my home. If I can keep it strong and efficient and pliable, I can only hope that it lasts for the full length of me.

But to *have* heart? I finally understand. The heart that cannot be tracked, measured, or monitored is the true epicenter of the self. It's the precise spot where the mind and body vie for a place of balance. Everything about me is constantly teetering, always searching for stillness, like the bubble bead inside a level. The heart remains constant while the mind and body change direction. Heart is neutrality and steadfastness. It's purity. It's a person's essence. It teaches about letting go to nothingness; therefore, it's everything. It's wisdom and kindness, acceptance and understanding, relief and integrity. It's desire and love, purpose and promise. I suppose it's my soul, the part of the infamous "mind-body-spirit" connection we seek. Something invisible, yet it's the one true thing we see and feel in everything we do.

Through fitness I learned how my mind and body could be in constant battle as well as perfect unity, but the place where it all levels out is the heart. Heart is where true strength lives. Fitness made me hardcore? Yes. And heart core? Definitely.

Funny how the heart is a muscle. The only one in the body that I can develop and train and still never truly see its progress through an impressive striation or aesthetic sweep. After all these years of fitness, I know it's strong the way a muscle can be, yet I feel its strength every single day in a completely different way. I try to identify what heart looks like, either very medical or something more ethereal, but it never leads to one thing. The sensations are present, though. The thumping. Beating. Racing. Slowing. I can feel it whooshing in my ears, pulsating inside my throat, living in my core. It activates when I push myself to a place that hurts a little to get to. It underscores parts of a journey that make me feel uncomfortable. As I try to breathe through the physical feeling and not mentally focus on any one thing, I get lost in the indescribable.

That's when I'm reminded: *Things are working out.*

FROM THE GYM BAG

THE NUMBERS

I've trained at approximately 40 different gyms in over 10 states, and that's including one-day passes at local gyms while traveling. The quantity of workouts astounds me— approximately 300 workouts per year, unless I was training split routines (one workout in the morning, one in the evening) for a bodybuilding competition, then that number basically doubles. So, that's a total of 18,600 workouts, which netted approximately 223,000 sets and an upward of 2.6 million total reps. I've lifted an aggregate of over 15 million pounds.

I've generated countless gallons of sweat, worn down hundreds of pairs of socks, turned the soles of dozens of pairs of sneakers to smooth rubbery bottoms, worn through a litany of workout clothing, gathered thousands of ponytails, rinsed hundreds of water bottles, washed dozens of commemorative T-shirts (like my pink Arnold Schwarzenegger T-shirt from Venice Beach), used hundreds of towels to wipe sweat, and listened to my "pump-up songs" hundreds of times.

Through counting, I was constantly at the precipice of a decision. I could either tell myself that I can't do this number, such as a set of 10, or I would commit to trying. I could set a goal of 10 reps, and when I was dying on rep seven, I had to either terminate the set or go in. Nine out of 10 times, I went in. Even when I knew, rationally, that going for a 350 deadlift on my third attempt in my first meet was completely ridiculous. (I got 310 the attempt right before. A 40-pound jump? Come on!) The success was always in the commitment to trying.

Oh, the number of times I've counted to eight, to 10, 12, 15, 25, 50—all in a single set. And then to do it again and again, all in the same session at the gym. All this counting offered up many opportunities to meditate against the digits.

When I count, I often look for the smallest fleck I can find in front of me to zero in on. A spot of black. A chip of paint. An irregular scuff on a wall ahead of me. A swirly electric green light shape inside the backs of my eyes after rubbing the sweat out of them. A thread on a sweatshirt. A number etched onto a weight. And mental mantras are like numbers: something simple I can always count on. Something I can fixate on in between the one and two and three and four. Lock into. A way of taking my mind from a googolplex of thought to an infinitesimal place.

THE GYMS

The gym has been my second home for a long time. It's the one place where I've always felt fully in my element (except for those early months when I didn't know what I was doing). Even now, I can walk into any gym, pretty much anywhere, and feel like I have every right to be there. Confidence through movement. The thing about being shaped by fitness for so long means I have established a comfortable relationship with these facilities that are often some of the strangest places on Earth. Because, very simply, gyms are like socially acceptable asylums. And I'm not casting judgment; I can be as quirky as the next guy. So many of us are intimidated by gyms, yet the people inside are usually the most accepting folks you'd ever meet. Gym membership meant I belonged, and as long as you pay your annual fee, you always do. Belonging comes with a right to be there, whether you're an expert or a novice. It's a qualification that doesn't come that easily in a divisive world.

Some of the many gyms I've belonged to include the Y, Diamond's Gym, Top This Gym, Mount Olympus Gym, and Bev Francis Gold's Gym. These were my New York stomping grounds. Once we moved to New Jersey, I found myself at the Y again, Pro Fitness Gym, Fitness Factory, New York Sports Club, Quest Gym, and Powerhouse Gym.

As much as I've loved being a part of each gym community, it's also a blast to cheat on your gym occasionally. A rogue workout at some faraway place, such as a day pass while on vacation or a new gym in town that just mailed you a free pass postcard, can be energizing. Some of those places have included Cape May Fitness, Planet Fitness, Anytime Fitness, Gold's Gym in Venice, Powerhouse Gym in Santa Monica, and Muscle Beach, Venice. I've also been seen at Dick's Sporting Goods testing out the elliptical cross trainers a bit too vigorously.

The names of the gyms are often as quirky as the people inside. But as crazy as the gym environment can be, it was where I've always felt most at home. The dingier the better; those I lovingly called a "hole in the wall" were my favorites. A grimy gym can be just as motivational as a sparkling new facility. You get the "underdog" feeling coursing through your veins.

When Craig and I bought our first home, one of our top criteria was to have an at-home gym in the basement. The basement walls and floors were unfinished, there was no heat or air conditioning, and cobwebs brushed our foreheads when descending the stairs; it was a dungeon, and that was perfect. As long as there were barbells and dumbbells, we were good to go.

In the two homes that we've lived in, we transformed the basement into a gym. In our first home, with the unfinished walls and low ceilings in the basement of our split-level home on Long Island, we crammed in as much iron as we could budget for. We shopped at garage sales for odds and ends to fill our space. In our present home, with a roomier unfinished basement with higher ceilings, we dragged the weights and machines from Long Island, and then supplemented our options over the years. When the movers brought us over the George Washington Bridge to our new home in New Jersey, they were faced with schlepping all the equipment downstairs—which included a rack of dumbbells from 10 to 85 pounds, plates ranging from 2½ pounds up to a stack of 45 pounds, flat bench press rack, power rack, leg press machine, leg extension machine (that converted to a leg curl), lat pull machine, and a variety of Bosu balls, jump ropes, and resistance bands. The staircase angle to the basement was sharp, thus the hole we made in the Sheetrock! It was quite the set-up, so much so that friends would come over to work out. While my preference has always been to train at a gym (I like the energy plus the range of equipment), it was critical to have options should there be a snowstorm or erratic schedule during which we wouldn't be able to get to the regular gym.

Gyms typically have mirrors. There's something about a room covered in mirrors, and filled with opportunities to better yourself, that makes you see who you are in both clear and distorted ways. It's all about tweaking what's on the outside, but when doing so, you can't help but affect what's under the hood. And isn't it ironic that every gym I've been to through the years has had cracks in the mirrors? Rumors were that someone tried to rack a weight and missed, or a brawl broke out. No one ever really knew how the cracks happened; they just seemed to show up the next day you were there. Whatever the case, gyms are the perfect place for self-examination. Of course, you wind up examining everyone else, too.

Because no matter the gym, there is always the same cast of characters. They are:

The screamers. (They are very loud when they work out.)

The beefcakes. (They have lots of brawn.)

The athletes. (They excel at everything.)

The nonathletes. (Aka the average Joes. They're doing their best.)

The powerlifters.

The bodybuilders.

The *David*s. (They have bodies that you can't stop staring at.)

The klutzes. (They drop stuff on themselves and on you.)

The procrastinators. (They spend a long time in the locker room or talking to you. Anything to avoid working out.)

The profuse sweaters. (They leave puddles wherever they go.)

The hoggers. (They use all the equipment and won't let you work in.)

The Monday nighters. (They come once per week, right after a weekend of partying too hard.)

The January-ers. (They make a New Year's resolution to exercise and then disappear the other 11 months of the year.)

The friends for life. (They are the people you meet at the gym who wind up becoming *your* people. Distance and time can't break those bonds. Once a fellow lifter, always a friend.)

The next generation. (They are the kids who are already working out and will probably do so for life.)

The courageous. (They are in the gym despite fear of looking dumb.)

The strong. (They just are.)

THE ACCESSORIES

Back in the day when I was getting hooked on exercise and needed motivation, guilt was my wearable. *Did I exercise today? Did I exercise enough? Did I push hard enough?* The questions weighed on me like a bench press. Guilt is a great driver for a slightly compulsive, hard-pushing person like me. These days, I'm committed to a wearable. It's my exercise shackle. If it looks like I'm in jeopardy of meeting my daily goals, my wearable zaps me. It's the tiniest, most effective training coach a person can have. Unless, of course, you forget to put it on or charge it. However, it has an attitude that I just don't appreciate sometimes. "Oh, hello" is my favorite message. It appears on the screen when I strap it on again in the morning. Attitude, as if I was supposed to have been up through the night jogging. Excuse me! I still hook it on each morning the second I get out of bed and take it off once I get into bed at night. (Don't want to lose out on any last steps going to the bathroom before bed.) I'm tethered to its beeping and pulsing and soft vibrations. My wearable gives me a better appreciation for what a dog feels when he dares to cross the invisible fence in the yard. But boy, it works. Behavior modification at its best.

It's hard to imagine life these days without a wearable, especially with the "sitting is the new smoking" thought tacked onto the bulletin board in my head. I'm a writer. I sit all day at the computer. So, what is that, a pack a day? Two packs when I'm cramming on a deadline? Studies support that even when we exercise for an hour each day, it doesn't necessarily offset all those other hours of sedentariness. I get a zap every so often that reminds me to move. It's *her* again, the stick figure attitude lady who waves her shapeless arms at me to take 240 steps. She might want to add a little bicep work to her repertoire. Still, I'm goal-oriented so when she asks, I listen. On days when I haven't reached my goal of 10,000 steps, you can find me running in place in my bathroom around 11:45 pm. *Can I do 2,500 steps in 15 minutes?* is not an uncommon thing for me to ponder at the closing hour of the day. My family yells at me to stop making noise, so I transfer my tapping feet to the bathmat by the shower. It's surprising how quickly you can rack up 1,000 steps just running in place. It's when I need to accumulate two or three thousand steps to hit the goal that I'm caught between extreme nighttime sports and defeat.

Whether the music was distracting me from the pain of pushing through another rep, or it was releasing a chemical in my brain that made me feel euphoric, tunes have always been a contributor to a workout well done.

One of the early pieces of workout paraphernalia that I owned was the Walkman. Prior to it, music was only present in the exterior environment. Whether it was piped in through the gym speakers or coming via the workout tape in the VCR, music was always a part of my workout. The big game changer came when the music went inside me. It's different when you are the only one listening to a song. It's personal. Sharing that song in a gym with all the other muscle heads works but not like this. You can increase the volume. You can change the song. You can replay it 10 times in a row without any judgment. It's your workout song.

With my Walkman, I could bring my favorite audio cassettes, like the full *90125* Yes album or Billy Joel's *Glass Houses*, on walks or runs and let the tunes lead the way. Some came with straps, so you could loop the entire thing over your neck and wear it like a necklace. (Not ideal for running; the unit banged across my chest with each sprint.) Too bad it didn't fit in my fanny pack! Flipping through the "B" side songs that I didn't like as much was difficult, too, but still, the Walkman was a novel tool for motivation. The Walkman progressed to one that could play CDs. The shape of the entire thing went from rectangular to round, but that didn't change any of the old problems. In fact, I found that a CD Walkman often skipped through songs if I was running. I guess that's why it was called a *Walk*-man. The headsets were cumbersome with large black foam pads sitting over my ears like earmuffs, both joined by a hardwire arch cradling the top of the head. It took quite a few years for the buds to shrink down enough to fit inside ears.

My first iPod Shuffle felt like I was holding a tiny miracle in my pocket. It was light and long, white and sleek, and I could pack in exactly 100 songs! Not just songs from one album, where the ones on the second side were just sort of *eh,* but the songs that I loved and wanted to hear again and again. Songs were 99 cents each, a tiny investment for a motivational fitness tool. This was a breakthrough for my workouts. It was also the beginning of a less patient me who now gives thumbs up and thumbs down to songs on Pandora like I'm giving out candy on Halloween. As the earbuds got smaller, the devices did, too—so small that they practically disappeared. Now I panic if I get to the gym and realize I left my earbuds home. I need them! They're not called "buds" for nothing.

Clothing accessories scrunched and slouched in the '90s. Scrunchies were oversized hair ties wrapped in fabric that I'd use to pull my hair back up into a ponytail. I had them in every color; some were velvet or chiffon, while others had bold patterns and bizarre prints. When my scrunchie wasn't in my hair, it was on my wrist. In that same decade, slouchy socks were all the rage. They looked like leg warmers but were thick cotton gym socks. They gathered around the ankles and came in all kinds of pastel colors like sea-foam green and peach.

The gym rat pack, particularly bodybuilders, wore big, baggy balloon pants (think MC Hammer pants) with wide elastic waistlines and cinched ankles. The patterns were loud, and the colors were vivid. Basically, hideous. The logos were obnoxiously gaudy, like a gorilla on steroids flexing his biceps. The sweatshirts had cut-off necklines to expose trap muscles and sayings such as "shut up and lift." My all-time favorite sweatshirt, which still lives in my closet, is a basic thick, plain gray. The cuffs and neckline are frayed, but it's still the little black dress of my fitness attire. It was a real find at five dollars at the Roosevelt Field Flea Market, circa 1989.

MOTIVATIONAL WORKOUT TIPS

I have my favorite workouts and "tricks" that have served me well throughout the years. Nothing here is backed by true fitness expertise, such as being a certified coach or having letters after my name. It's just me sharing personal experiences and hoping that something here can work for you, too.

Let's start with the easiest tip of all: move your body 7 days a week. It doesn't have to be all-out efforts each time or anything fancy or overly formal. Plain old motion instead of still. Just by breathing you're in motion. Now, all you have to do is add a little commotion to the motion. Park in the far, unfavorable spots in the parking lot. Avoid the moving walkway at the airport. Pace around your house while you're on a phone call and suddenly you've walked a quarter of a mile. Instead of eating lunch at your desk, mindlessly scrolling on your phone, take 10 slow laps around your floor and *then* eat your lunch. (You won't get sweaty, but your blood will circulate.) If you're stuck in the car a lot, you can contract and release your abdominals at every red light to tighten your core. Move, move, move.

With that said, if it's in the budget, get a wearable device and wear it. Strive for a set number of steps each day and preprogram it into your device. My goal is 10,000 daily steps, which is approximately five miles. A wearable is like a 24/7 workout partner. It'll hold you accountable, nudge and cheer you, and help you reach your goals. With many of us working at desks all day or driving in cars, it's way too easy to not feed our bodies the gift of movement. A clever option to a wearable is to find an app that can send get-up-and-move alerts to your smartphone to turn it into an all-day pedometer. If you don't have a smartphone, just resort to an old-fashioned clock.

Pick your pump-up song. What's the one song right now that gets you so jazzed up that you feel like dancing around the house and singing at the top of your lungs? The song that pumps you up to the point where you are 1,000 percent sure you could leap over the neighbor's fence? The song that you would want to break a finish line ribbon with? *This* is your pump-up song. Keep it readily at your fingertips so you can play it on the drive to the gym or when you're about to swipe your gym card and feel the intimidation factor closing in on you. We all deserve our own Rocky bolting up the Philadelphia Museum of Art stairs song. Your pump-up song is the one that, no matter how many times you hear it, gets you psyched. Play it a lot.

Pick your mantra. We all talk to ourselves, even if it's just via the dialogue we keep privately in our heads. Too often that dialogue is uninspiring or hurtful. When negativity creeps in and the *can't's* dominate your thoughts, reach for your mantra. Let it be positive. Let it be kind. Imagine it being the most encouraging thing you would tell your best friend who is doubting his or her ability. *You can do anything. You are so strong. Keep up the great work. You're a survivor.* Something that resonates with you. Then actually speak it—say it out loud, shout it out in the shower, start your day by putting it out to the Universe, then give it back to yourself right before you go to sleep. Like your song, this mantra can change daily or never. There's no right or wrong as long as you're honoring what you need at that moment in time.

Always believe in yourself. The positive dialogue inside your head should always win out in the "good and evil" self-thoughts battle. Remind yourself over and over again that you are capable of everything and anything you set your sights on. Even when believing in yourself seems illogical, do it anyway.

Sign up for something and go public with it. Set a goal. Make it tiny, like "I'm going to the gym today," and then tell someone. Text your friend, and even tell her to ask you later about the workout. Or go bigger, like compete or participate in something. A race, a walk, a bodybuilding show—anything you can use as an excuse to reach a fitness goal. When you've attached your name to something and posted it on social media, your pride is on the line. No one wants to feel like a quitter in front of all those followers.

Then wait one week before you "quit" anything. Maybe you made it to the gym one night or you took a spin class, but you're not motivated to go back. Is it because it physically hurt? Bruised your ego because you felt self-conscious and embarrassed? Were you just bored? The point is, you need to give yourself a chance for fitness to catch. *Hang in there.* Keep moving through your process until you find what you love— or at least like enough to show up again. And again. Fitness is more about what you do, not what you don't do. So, actually, *don't* wait a week to quit—just keep going.

Practice being comfortable with uncomfortable. When you work at establishing your own connection with fitness, you're going to feel discomfort along the way. Your muscles, joints, ego, and pride are all tender areas that will feel the impact of your fitness journey. You're either going to feel discomfort while you're in the midst of exercise (like that stitch in your side from running) or 24–72 hours after exercise (DOMS: delayed onset muscle soreness that makes it impossible to sit down without pain) or before exercise (when you feel like a fish out of water at the gym). If you're working your body hard, there's no way around it. I say acknowledge the hurt. Expect it, even. So, when it shows up (and it always does), your mind will have the confidence to out-power it. *You're almost there.* This mantra has sustained me through the push portion of an all-out sprint or a last rep. The discomfort that the body is feeling triggers the mind, and that is what topples well-intended gym members. However, the more you can push yourself through unfavorable feelings of a stitch or winded lung or an embarrassment, the more unstoppable you become.

Accept that you are going to look and feel dumb at some point. I've literally flown off of a treadmill at the gym. Back in the day, the guys at Diamond's Gym would laugh at me when I did heavy squats because, with each rep, I made the sound,

"Shoop!" I get sweat stains that make me look like I peed my pants. Unwelcome farts, burps, and buggers are inevitable. Who cares? When you work your body, weird stuff is bound to happen. Laugh it off.

Weed out your Pattys. If anyone in your life is counting your tummy rolls, tell them to hit the road. We have no time to belittle the skin we are in right now. Pay close attention to those who might be hijacking your exercise goals, too. Tempting you with baked goods when they know you're trying to eat a cleaner diet is not supportive. Call them out on this behavior because, chances are, they are not even aware of what they're doing.

Find a workout partner. Someone who pushes you to be your best, and someone you can push right back. Who knows, you might wind up marrying each other. Or maybe you already did!

Revisit your favorite childhood sneakers. Chances are, they're back in style after all these decades. When you put them on, you'll be whisked back in time with a little extra pop in your step.

Utilize the gym that comes with your present routine. If you're in high school, college, or graduate school, you probably have access to some amazing gym facilities. It's part of the tuition or your taxes, so get your money's worth. If there's a gym at the office and it's free to employees, get down there during lunch or before work. The convenience of these workout facilities, whether it be by location or price, can aid in finding your fitness consistency.

Make peace with the mirrors. They reflect so much, yet so little. Take them for what they are—a chance to see the shell as it is right now. If you spot something that makes you cringe or become self-critical, shift your emphasis to the positive. Your powerful legs, your head-to-toe being, the environment around you. Or just reposition your thoughts to a place of nonjudgment and neutrality: "What do I see? I see a woman and she is smiling at me."

Focus on your own mat. It's way too easy to compare how your warrior pose looks against the guy in front of you. But the truth is, it just doesn't matter. OK, maybe it does if you're competing in bodybuilding or trying to place in a marathon. But for the most part, putting the blinders on and just doing your own thing is the best way to dive deep into your own strength.

Wipe your sweat. No one likes sitting on a drippy machine at the gym, so be sure to clean things off after your turn. Follow gym etiquette such as racking your weights after you use them (it's comparable to pushing in your chair at the dinner table), not walking inches in front of someone while they're lifting (would you make funny faces at someone while they're taking a serious call?) and letting people *work in* if they ask (meaning, don't hog machines). Fitness can be all about you, but at the same time, being in a gym reminds us that we're part of a greater community of like-minded, dedicated peeps. Respecting the tools, space, and people within the four walls builds respect for oneself, too.

Embrace that anyone can get into fitness at any time in life. Even if you've always been the most nonathletic, two-left-footed person, you can still make exercise a part of your life. If you're at an age where you're thinking *Why start now?* flip the thought to *Why not start now? Now* is always the perfect time to kickstart anything that can enrich your life and help you grow as a person.

Cultivate your strength. This is the big one. Committing yourself to consistent fitness is a great way to reinforce just how strong you can be. Commitment in itself is a sign of strength. Accepting the times when we falter is also indicative of strength. If you fumble, so be it. Just get back on track. It's like taking a trolley ride in San Francisco. On and off, on and off. Sometimes that's the fun of it because you pick up new experiences along the way for the next leg of the journey. When you build your body's physical strength through exercise, you impact the control center of yourself. *Where does strength come from?* Within.

THE WORKOUT ROUTINES

The following workouts were my go-to's throughout the years. They were the bones for the routines I built while bodybuilding as well as exercising for just general fitness. Designed to challenge the entire body each week by working different body parts at a time, these exercises can be bundled together in a myriad of ways. For example, if you go to the gym Monday, Wednesday, and Friday, you can pair up body parts to work together. Monday might be a chest and back workout, or what we gym rats call a "push/pull" workout. (Push is the predominant movement for the chest exercises, as in pushing things off your chest; pull is the opposite for the back, such as lat pulls.) Wednesday can be arms and shoulders. Friday can be a leg day. Abs can be peppered into every workout. Cardio, such as running or brisk walking or whatever you like to do to raise your heart rate, can be inserted any day.

Let your fitness choices help you achieve your goals. If you want to build more muscle mass, keep the weights heavier and the reps lower. If you're interested in toning, the weights can be lighter as the reps increase. As a believer in weight-bearing exercise for muscle strength and bone density, especially for women, I'm a proponent of incorporating "iron" in the diet. You can also use your own body weight to create resistance, build strength, and increase flexibility. Push-ups, pull-ups, planks, burpees, wall sits, lunges, single leg deadlifts (these are also great for balance), squats (using just your own body weight), tuck jumps, and calf raises are just a few of many exercises you can do anywhere, anytime. So easy and so effective!

Maybe you're trapped inside the house due to inclement weather. Or you have to travel and there's no gym in sight. Motion can still commence. Turn your body and the little space you might have around you into a makeshift workout arena. At the very least, march in place. Before you know it, you'll accumulate enough steps to reach your daily goal. There's tons of how-to articles, videos, and apps to walk you through all types of workouts. If any of this sounds overwhelming, start with an exploration of one exercise. *Just one step.*

Exercise smartly by consulting with your physician and by getting guidance from certified trainers.

Abs (Abdominals)

1–7 days per week

10–200 reps each time

The 10 reps mean you can start slow and small and build over time. You can make quick progress with ab exercises if you chunk them down into sizable amounts and keep building. Do two sets of 10 the first day, next day three sets of 10, and so on. Rep by rep. Build, build, build.

Engage your core every single day, whenever you can. Pay attention to your posture and activate your core (it will feel like a core when it's engaged, a tummy when it's not!). Core also equals your back, so you need to lift, and bend smartly, plus stretch and strengthen your back. Don't cheat. No swinging your body for momentum, no neck craning to hurl your shoulders off the floor when crunching. Take your time with each rep. Better to squeeze your abs hard each time and hold the squeeze for two or three seconds than to rush through it. It's not a race.

My favorite exercises:

- Planks
- Kettlebell swings
- Crunches
- Bicycles
- Scissors
- V-ups
- Ball work

Chest (Pecs)

1–2 times per week

8–12 sets total, 10–15 reps each

My favorite exercises:

- Bench press (flat bench and/or incline bench)
- Dumbbell press (flat bench and/or incline bench)
- Pec machine
- Push-ups (slow and steady wins the race with this exercise. You may need to start with knees on the floor, but over time, you will get stronger. Be patient and consistent.)
- Dips

Back (Lats)

1–2 times per week

8–12 sets total, 10–15 reps each

My favorite exercises:

- Lat pulls
- Dumbbell rows
- Deadlifts
- Pulls-ups and/or chins (for most women they might seem utterly impossible at first, because they are, but this is another slow and steady exercise that you can conquer if you just keep at it. Ask your workout partner to spot you until the day you do one rep on your own. It will happen!)

Shoulders (Delts)

1–2 times per week

8–12 sets total, 10–15 reps each

My favorite exercises:

- Dumbbell overhead press
- Front dumbbell raises
- Side lateral dumbbell raises
- Rear dumbbell flies
- Upright rows
- Shrugs

Arms (Bi's, aka Guns, and Tri's)

1–2 times per week

8–12 sets total, 10–15 reps each

My favorite exercises:

Biceps

- Dumbbell curls
- Barbell curls
- Killer 21s (7 bottom-half reps, 7 top-half reps, 7 full-range reps)
- Hammer curls
- Concentration curls

Triceps

- Overhead dumbbell extensions
- Dumbbell kickbacks
- Cable extensions
- French curls (skull crushers)

Legs (Quads, Hammies, Glutes, Calves)

1–2 times per week

8–12 sets total, 10–15 reps each

My favorite exercises:

- Squats (dumbbell or barbell)
- Step-ups
- Lunges
- Jump squats
- Leg curls
- Leg extensions
- Deadlifts
- Stiff-leg deadlifts
- Wall sits
- Toe raises

TIPS FOR AVOIDING GYM INTIMIDATION

Imagine a tool box filled with every kind of screw, nail, nut, and bolt that exists. There's hardware all over the place! But what if you don't know your Phillips heads from your washers, your ¾" screw from your 1¾"? In the calm, rational section of your brain, you recognize that these pieces can assist you in building something. However, in the gray matter where panic is taking flight, you don't know where to begin. That's what it can feel like when walking into a gym.

There are complicated machines everywhere, people who look like they know what they're doing, and you. The instinct might be to turn around and walk out the door. The better choice is to stay put and do something.

Whether you're walking into a gym you've just joined, a gym you joined but never go to, or a gym you're testing out, here are eight easy steps for giving you the guts to not run away:

1. **Find a treadmill.** It's the most basic, recognizable, and uncomplicated piece of cardio equipment available to mankind. Walk with confidence to that treadmill. Get on it. Press start and just put one foot in front of the other. Simple. Do this for 5–10 minutes while you warm up your body and strategize your next 50 minutes. Or continue walking for 20–30 minutes, upping the speed as you go for a cardio

workout. Walking on a treadmill is a great stall tactic and confidence builder, plus you can get a really good workout on it.

2. **Identify a location.** It's like walking into a cocktail party and deciding where you're going to stand. Grab a bench or find a spot off to the side away from people whose intensity is freaking you out. Claim it as your space for the next few minutes.

3. **Grab a pair of dumbbells.** Make sure the weights match (as in both weigh 10 pounds) and that they're not too heavy. If you're just starting out or warming up, err on the lighter side. The weights should feel like you're carrying two bags of groceries, not two bags of mulch. Exercise machines can be tricky with all the seat and bar adjustments. If you don't finagle them right, you can have poor alignment and ultimately hurt yourself. If you're feeling too shy to ask someone who works at the gym to help you, go straight to the iron. The iron is your friend.

4. **Move those dumbbells.** Do what I did at 16 years old when my dad gave me my dumbbells. Curl them, press them. Focus on moving slowly and with good form. Key into how the repetitions make your body feel. (Not sure what good form is? See number six.)

5. **Focus on numbers.** To avoid feeling like the world is staring at you, get lost inside your counting. Fifteen repetitions each time you do a set. Three sets. Hold a plank for 30 seconds. When you count, you also breathe, which is a good thing. The rhythmic count is meditative, too. Recite your personal mantra, again and again until you believe it. Repetition is practice, and practice makes perfect.

6. **Push yourself to ask for help.** Once you're over the hump of self-doubt and embarrassment, ask a trainer for assistance on how to work certain machines or to confirm your form on a movement. (Or ask for assistance to actually move you *over* the hump.) Many gyms offer a free training session with membership. Make it about you getting information, because information equals power.

7. **Quiet the voice in your head that's messing with you.** Whether you're in or out of the gym, your head will be working overtime, all the time, to make you doubt yourself and your ability to actually stick with a fitness plan. Patty from dance class was still counting my rolls years after I quit dance. Replace that dialogue with kindness and your pump-up songs. One of mine is still Joan Jett's "Bad Reputation." There's something about the beat that brings out my inner beast, especially at the beginning where it sounds like a jacked-up Slinky about to explode. Pump-up songs are like jumper cables. Everyone should have them in the trunk.

8. **Now do it again.** No matter how good or bad all that felt, don't dwell on it. Just do it again. Motion approved.

FINAL THOUGHTS

If you've been contemplating getting into fitness, but it just hasn't clicked yet for you, remember *you are already in motion*. The fact that you are alive, you are breathing, and you have things to do each day classifies you as active. Even in sleep we are in motion. The eyes flutter, the chest rises and falls, the body moves about, and the mind runs its course in dreams. Inactive is when we power down. Still. Done.

So, if you accept this "motion notion," and that being active is not something that you aspire to be *one day* but are already doing (maybe you just want to be *more* active), then the best thing is to keep moving. If exercising is one of your goals, whether it be adding it or maintaining it, take your already active body and move it in the direction of people, places, things—these are your tools—that you can grab onto to propel your fitness forward.

If you're willing to remove the labels from your being (e.g., inactive, not active enough, couch potato), then you're open-minded enough to close off any thoughts that stop your motion. *I'm too busy today. I'll start tomorrow. What's the point? This is too hard. I can't.*

Oh, yes you can.

Put your feet in charge. Keep stepping forward. Left, right, left, right. Lose yourself in the rhythm of one, two, one, two as you step out of the car and walk into the gym, walk onto a treadmill, walk, walk off the treadmill, walk over to the dumbbells, pick up a pair, and let your arms take over so your feet can rest. One, two, one, two. Curl those dumbbells until you've done a set or two or five. Walk over to another machine. Sit on it. Pull or push something. Motion, motion. By now you're feeling more than active; you're feeling alive. Your mind is desperately trying to walk you out of doing your physical actions, but your physical motion is too perpetual to allow for anything to break through. Walk back to the treadmill, a little faster this time, and walk some more, maybe even more briskly, or possibly move in a slow jog or a run or even a sprint. Walk it off for a few minutes as you cool down. Walk over to the stretching area. Move your body down to the floor. Move the upper half up and down, over and over, as you engage your abdominals. Motion, motion. Walk back to the car and motion onto your next thing that day. Now you can let your mind have its turn, but it's probably too embarrassed to say something dumb, like "You hate the gym, don't you?" Because you don't. The gym is merely the place. It's the act of motion that you love or are learning to embrace.

Maybe we make fitness more complicated than it needs to be. And maybe we do this as a distraction, so we don't have to put in the hard work. But our bodies are built for hard work. The complexity of our every system, from the cardiovascular to the skeletal, is designed for effort. You wouldn't purchase a new car with a powerful engine and leave it idle in the garage for 85 years. Just keep moving. It's that simple.

Competitive bodybuilding was the time in my life that underscored how much fitness and food could work together for a greater good. The countless hours of physical training would not have resulted in the best gains if I was putting the wrong nutrients in my body. Exercise broke down my body; good proteins and clean eating helped to repair it and build it up. What we do with our bodies and what we put inside our bodies can work hand in hand in driving our fitness efforts forward. But we all know this already!

However, it's way too easy for these two tracks to work independently of each other. My father epitomized the disconnect between exercise and eating. He may have been committed to his weight training for years, but he couldn't align that passion with healthy eating habits.

We all have personal traditions around food, both good and bad. Food is often triggered by events and emotions. We use it to soothe, celebrate, satiate, nourish. Intellectually, we understand what's healthy and what's not. Things can get messy.

My main tip for finding your elixir with healthy eating is to just keep moving your body. Every single day. Make it that simple. Let go of the mindset of *If I fail with one, why bother with the other?* While you're in motion, and remember you are already doing that just by breathing every day, tweak what you do around food. Swap out one habit one day for one different idea. For example, tomorrow, try flip-flopping your meals around. Eat like a king for breakfast (your largest meal of the day, which is typically dinner), like a prince for lunch (your medium-sized meal of the day), and then like a pauper for dinner (your smallest meal of the day, which is usually breakfast). This experiment puts all your calories in place for the work ahead of you for the day, not after the fact when you're just sitting around at night watching TV. Forgo shaking extra salt on your food before you even taste it. And then, when you do taste the eggs and they're super-bland, remind yourself it's OK to *be comfortable with uncomfortable.* Eat the eggs this time without the salt. See what happens if you walk yourself through that one simple act. This is how we start to retrain our thoughts and taste buds and create change. In time, you might find that your body will start craving more of the good stuff to help in making it strong.

Why is it that little kids love to run around? Why do they love to do funny things with their bodies, like hanging upside down or jumping on your bed or spinning in circles? It's because it's natural to move our bodies. We're built for it. Plus, it's fun! We teach ourselves to be sedentary and our bodies, the well-trained, intricate machines that they are, comply.

Bottom line: just start exercising.

That's my advice.

Stop contemplating it. Take one simple step today. Right now. Walk briskly around your kitchen for five minutes. Next time, six minutes. Then seven. We're all getting older so today is the day to get started. Remember that running water can't freeze.

If you're already working out, keep up the good work. Push yourself a little past what you thought was your best. Set big or little goals and knock them down with power.

You can be stronger than you think.

FROM THE PHOTO ALBUM

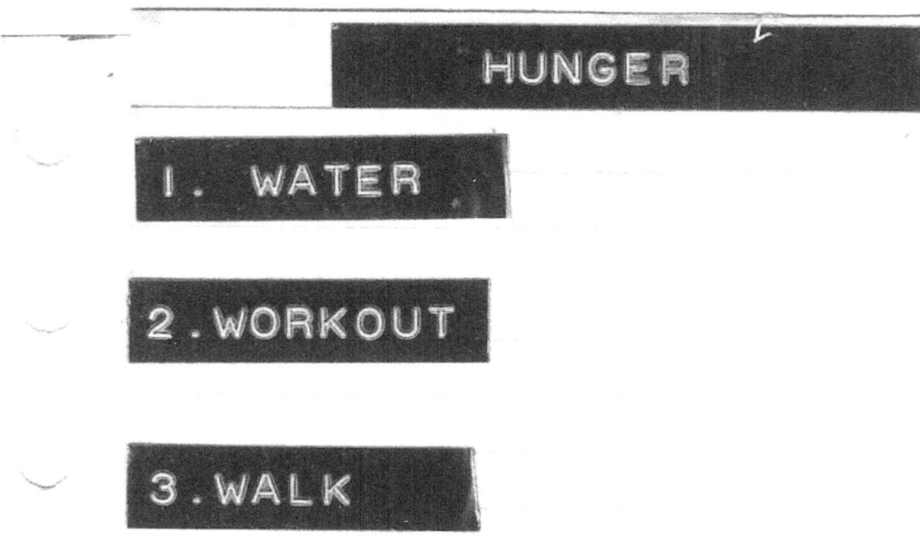

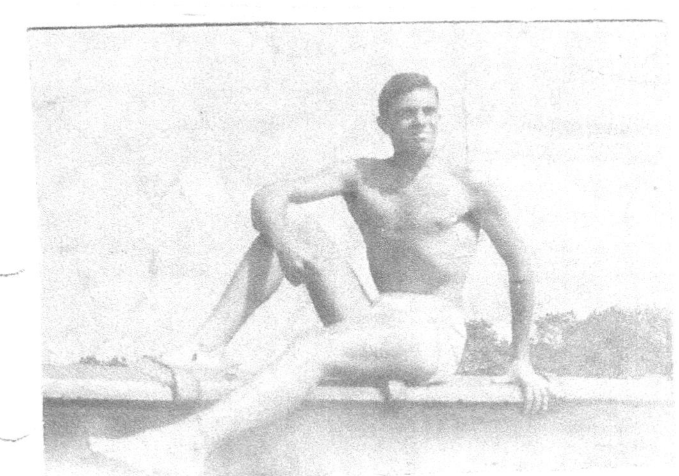

First page from Dad's little black workout book. Words to live by and an inspiring photo of himself as a young man.

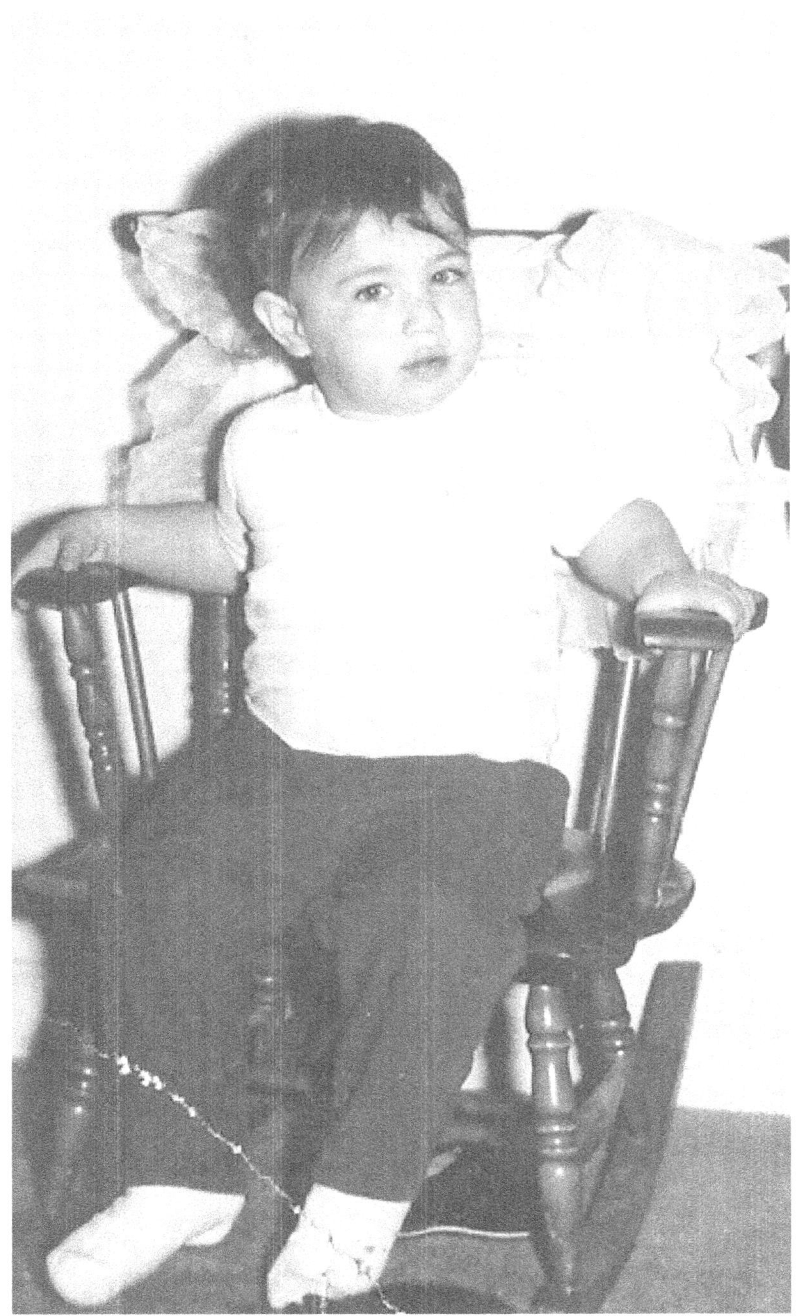

Little "HercuLisa."

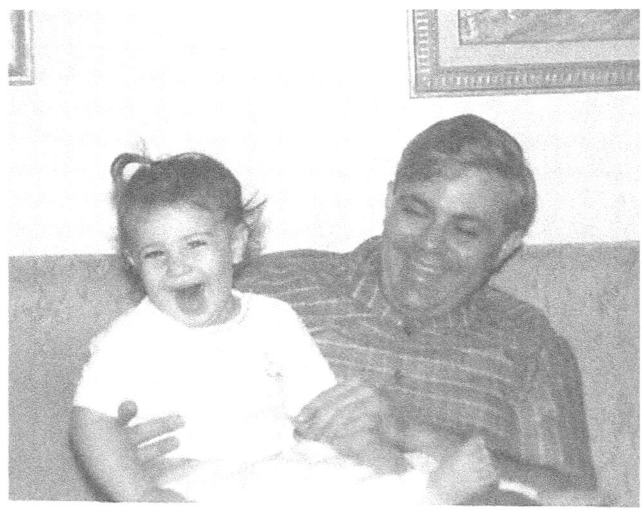

Dad looking like the teddy bear I grew up with.

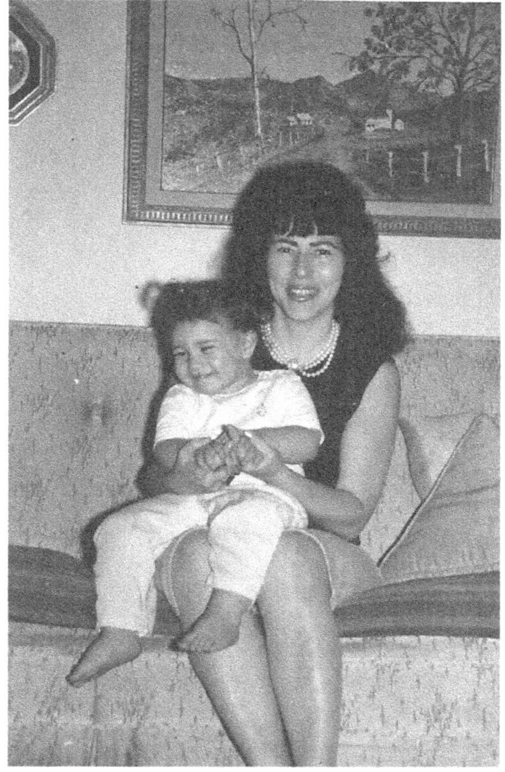

Mom always looking glam.

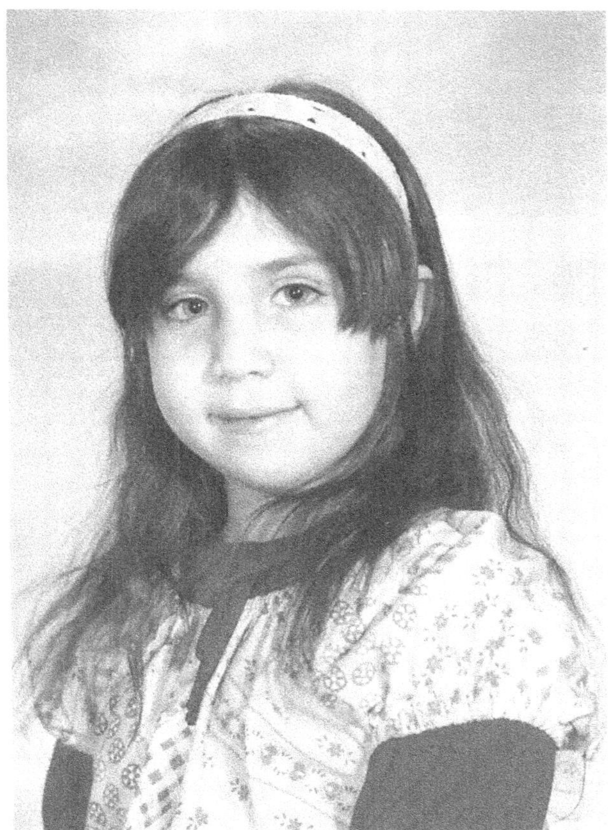

From the early dance years.

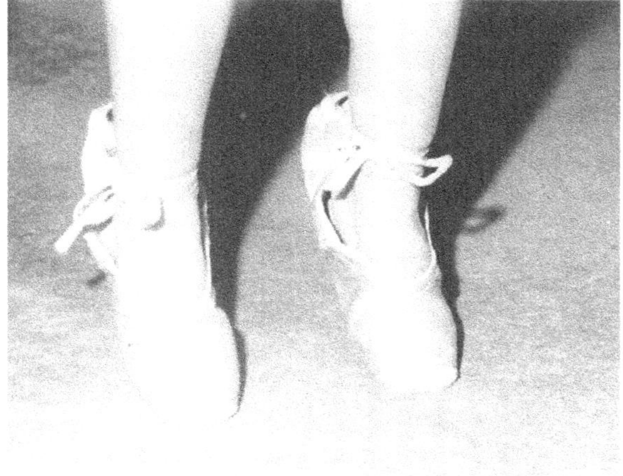

Dancing *en pointe* in Grandma's old ballet slippers
until, one day, I'd have my own.

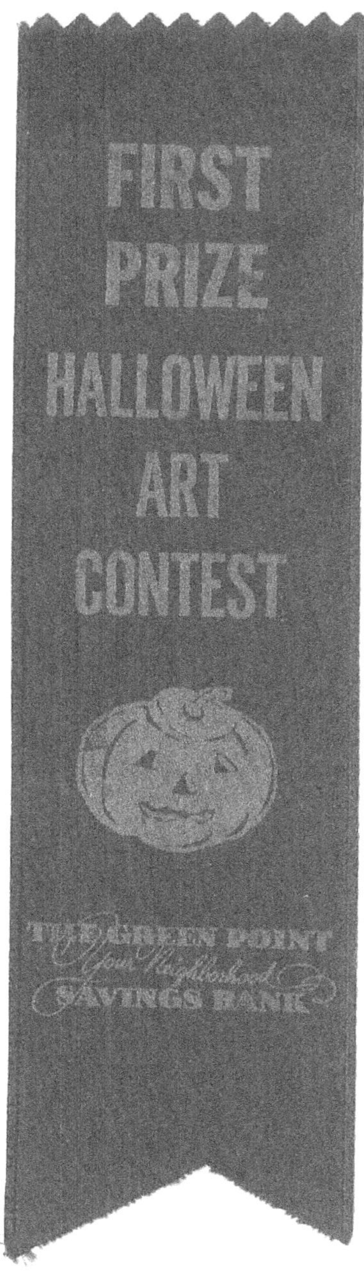

First "win" ribbon from the Halloween art contest!

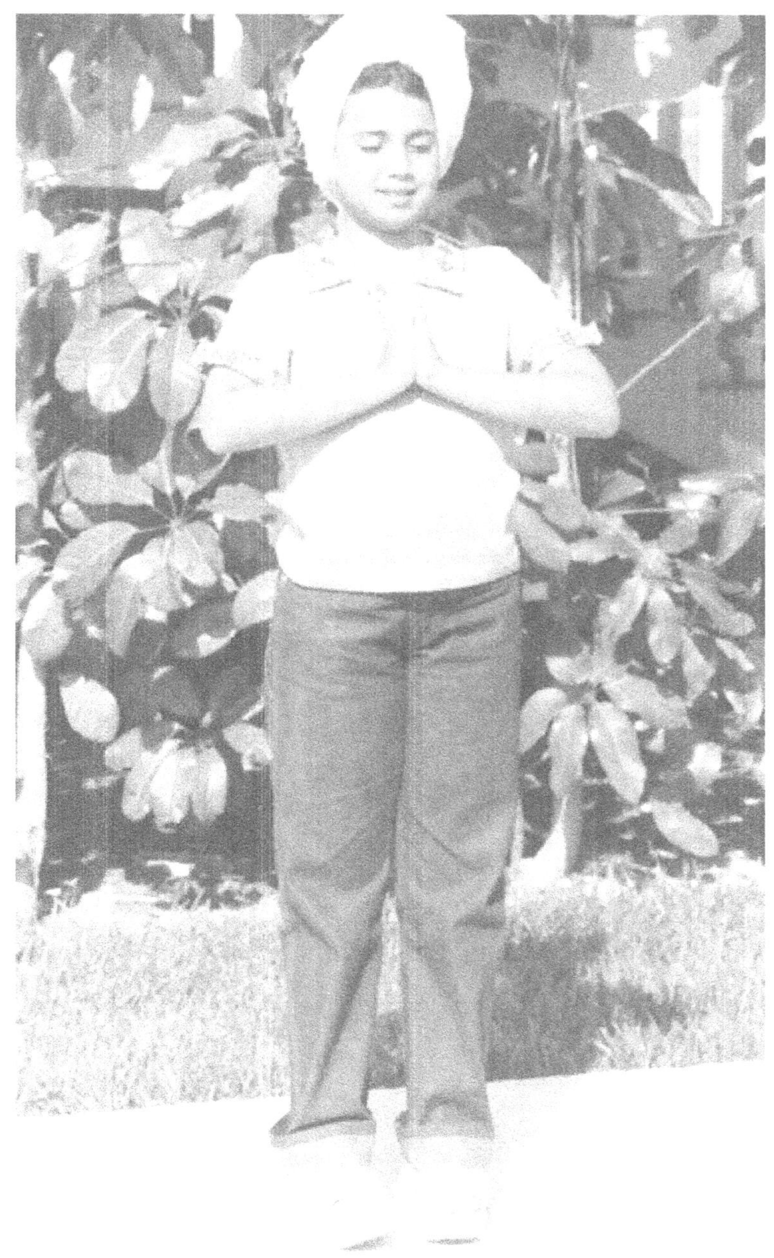

Learning about yoga during summer trips
to Grandma and Grandpa's in Florida.

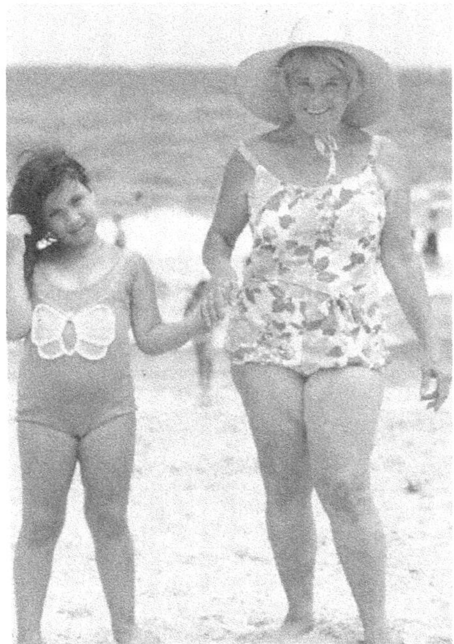

At the beach with Grandma.

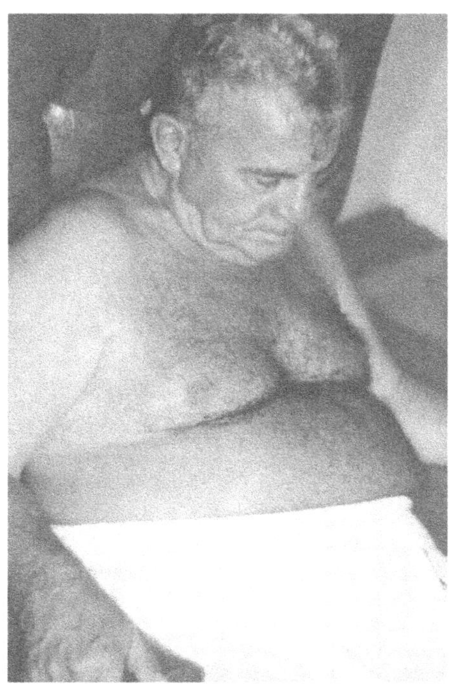

Grandpa, resting after backyard belly bumps.

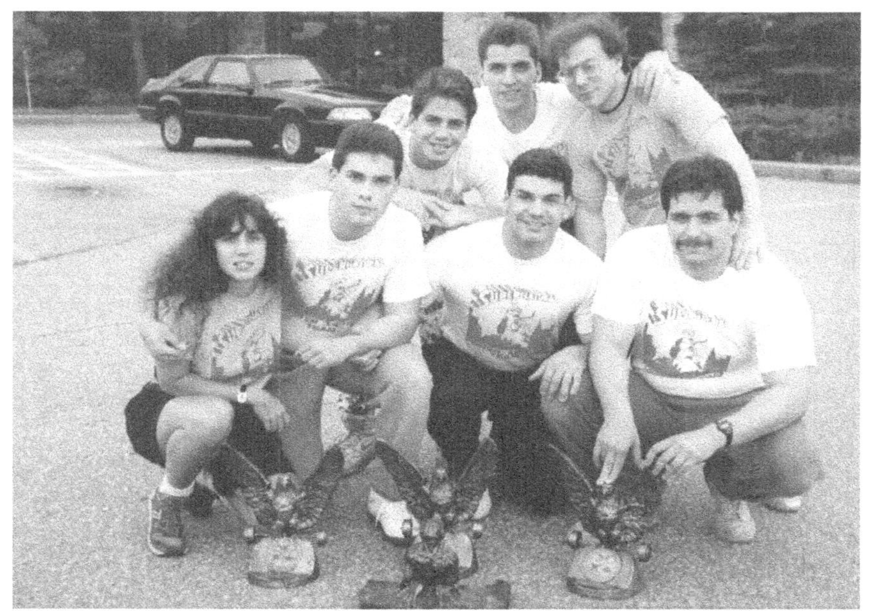

With the powerlifting team after a meet.

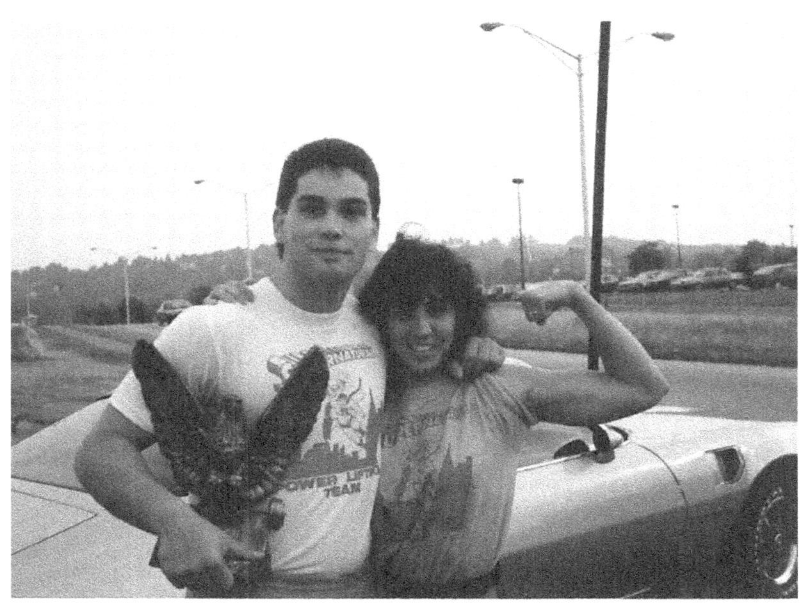

With my workout (and life) partner, Craig, after the meet.
The eagle trophy (which was made of concrete)
weighed more than the weights we lifted!

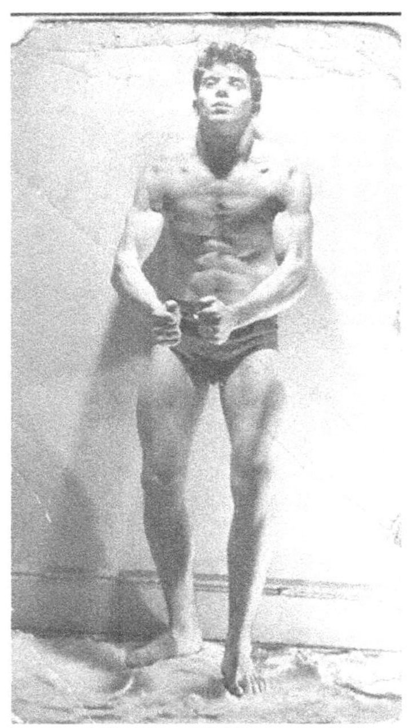

Uncle Steve hitting the "most muscular" pose.

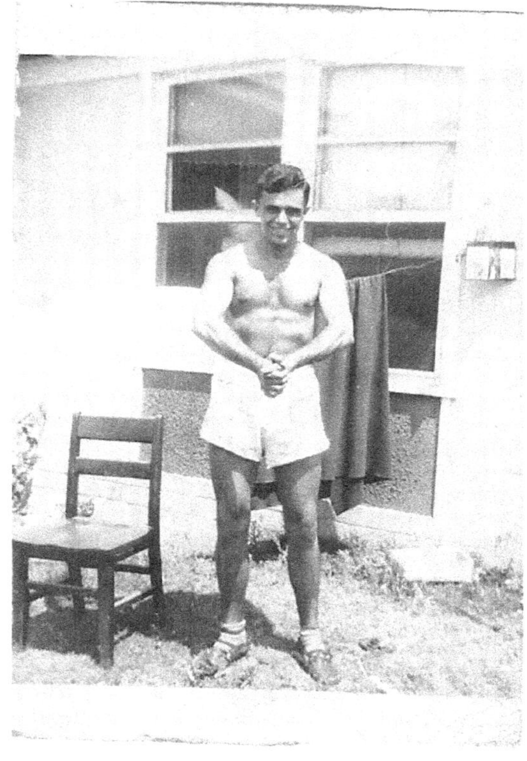

Dad's "most muscular."

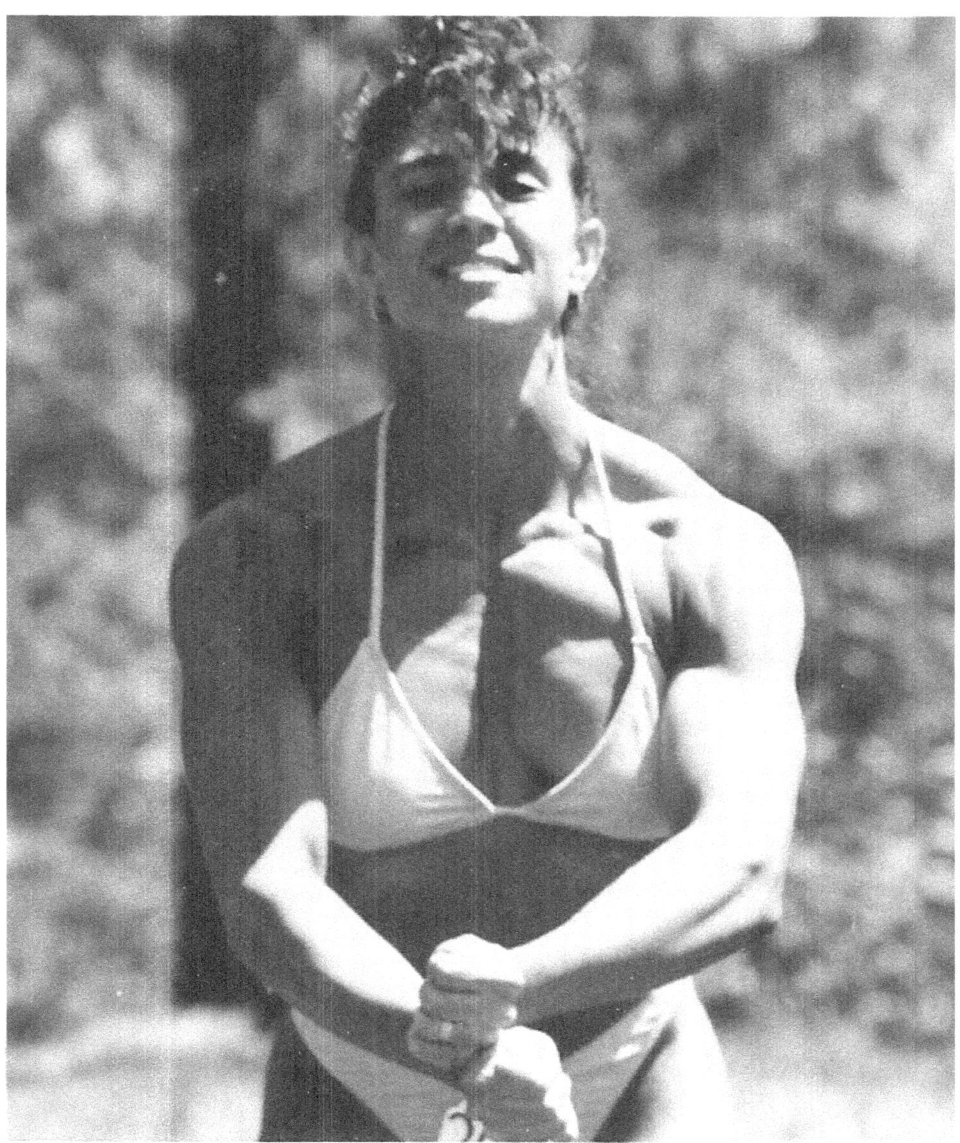

"Most muscular" pose ... it runs in the family.

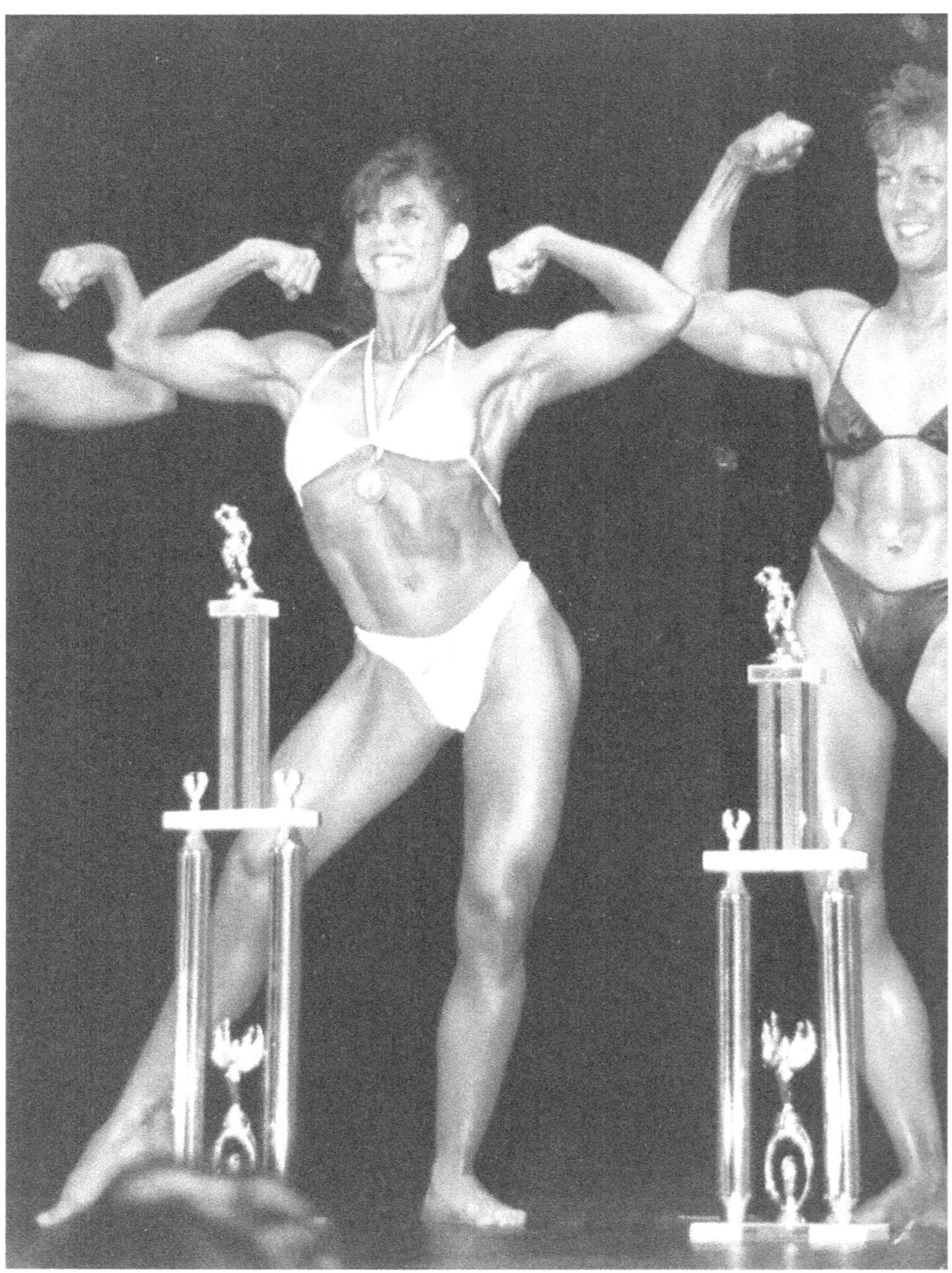

First bodybuilding competition, first place.

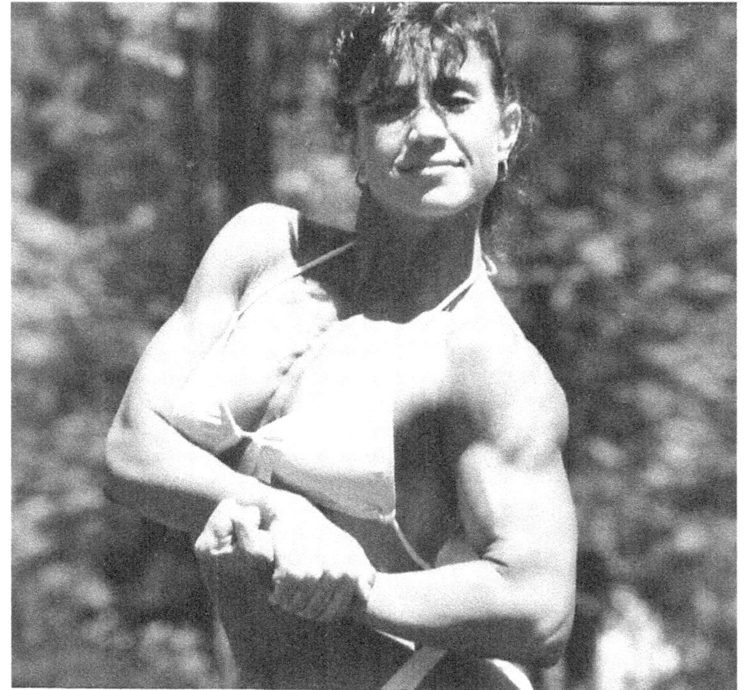

Side chest pose.

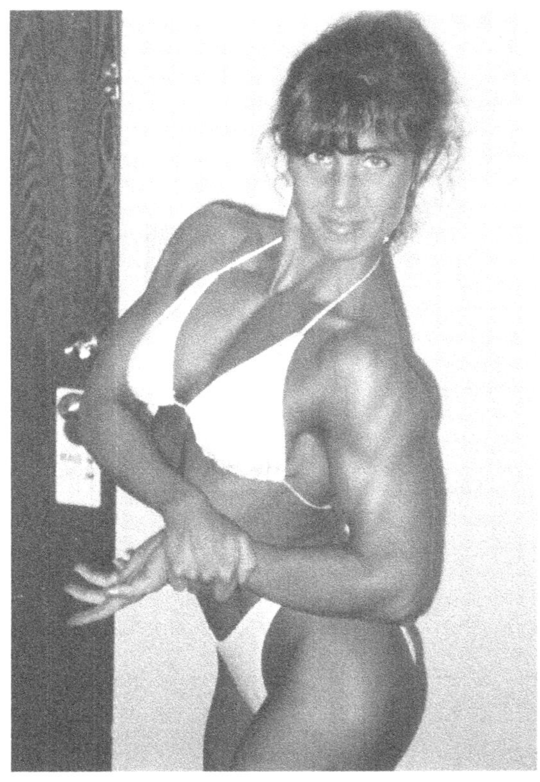

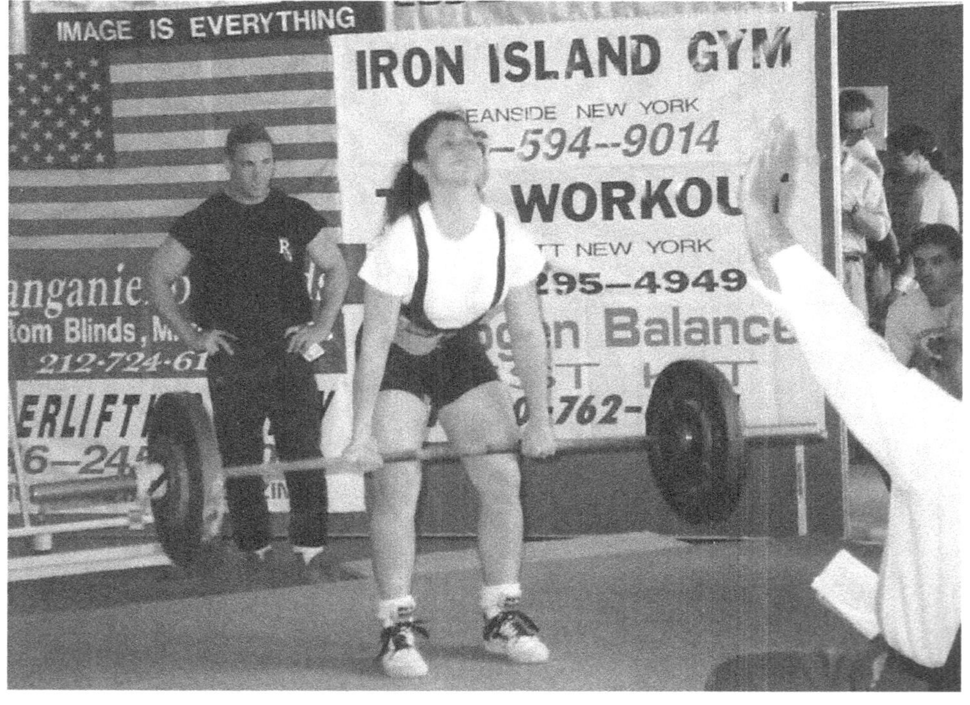

Pulling up a deadlift, conventional style, in a powerlifting meet.

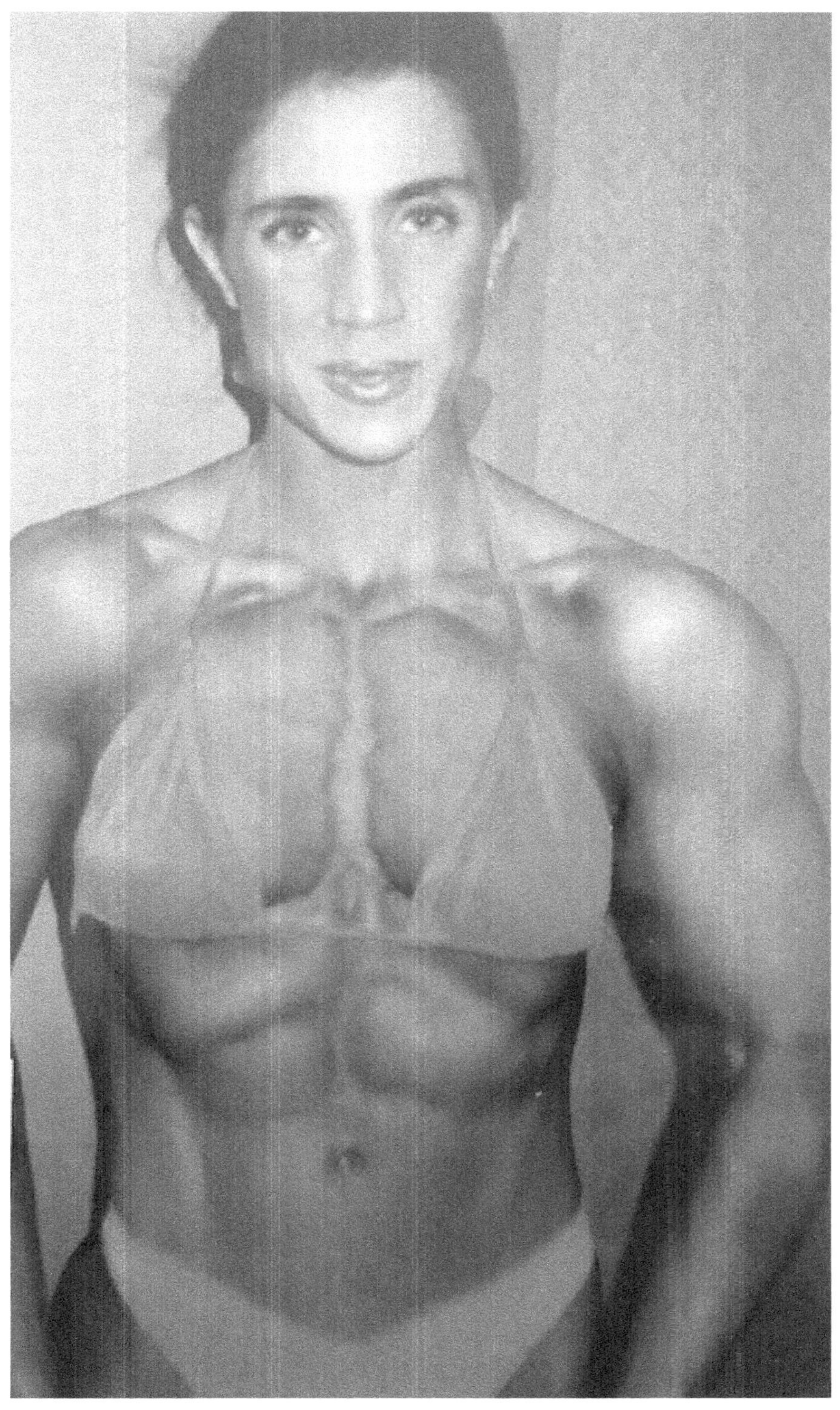

On the day of a pro bodybuilding competition. Ripped, tan, oiled, and dying for pizza.

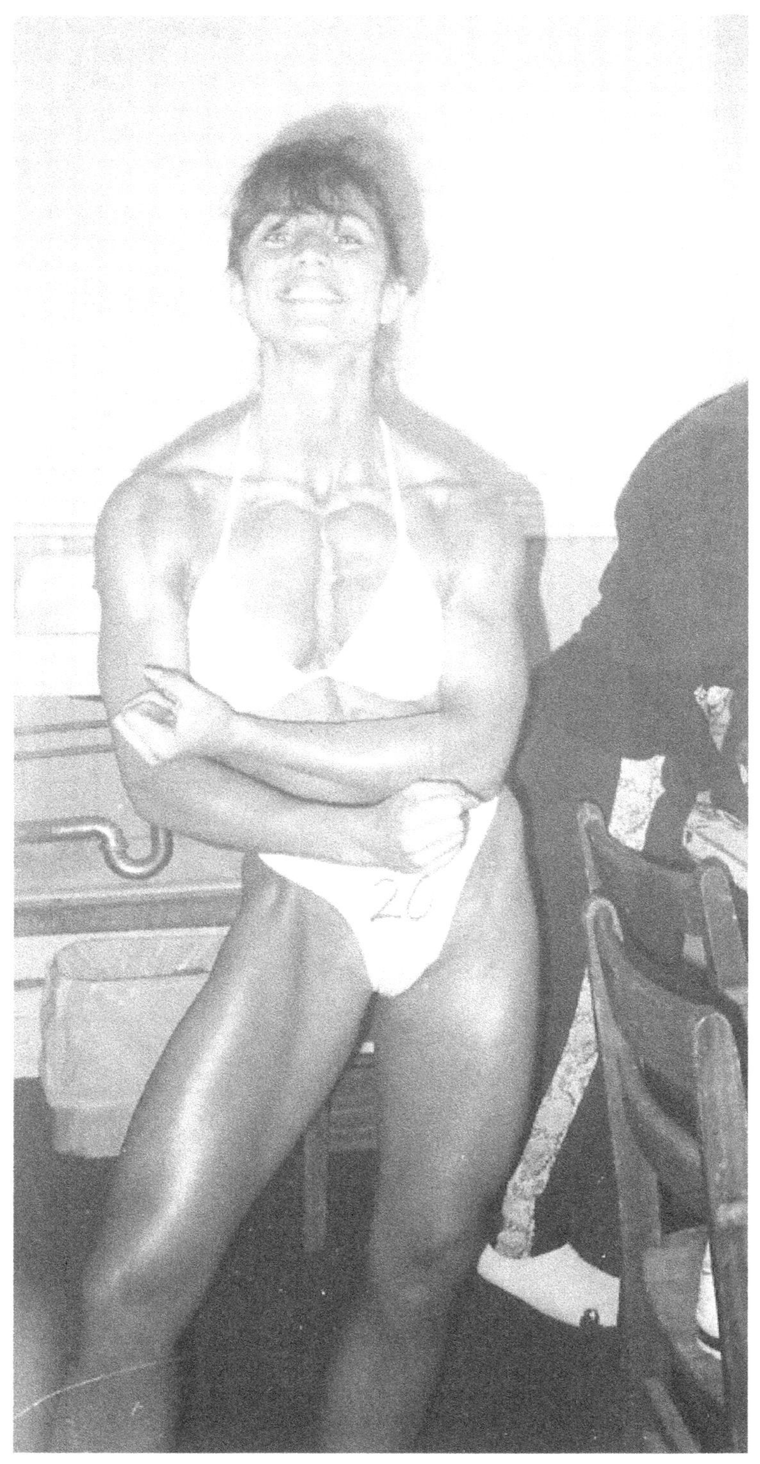

Pumping up backstage before a show.

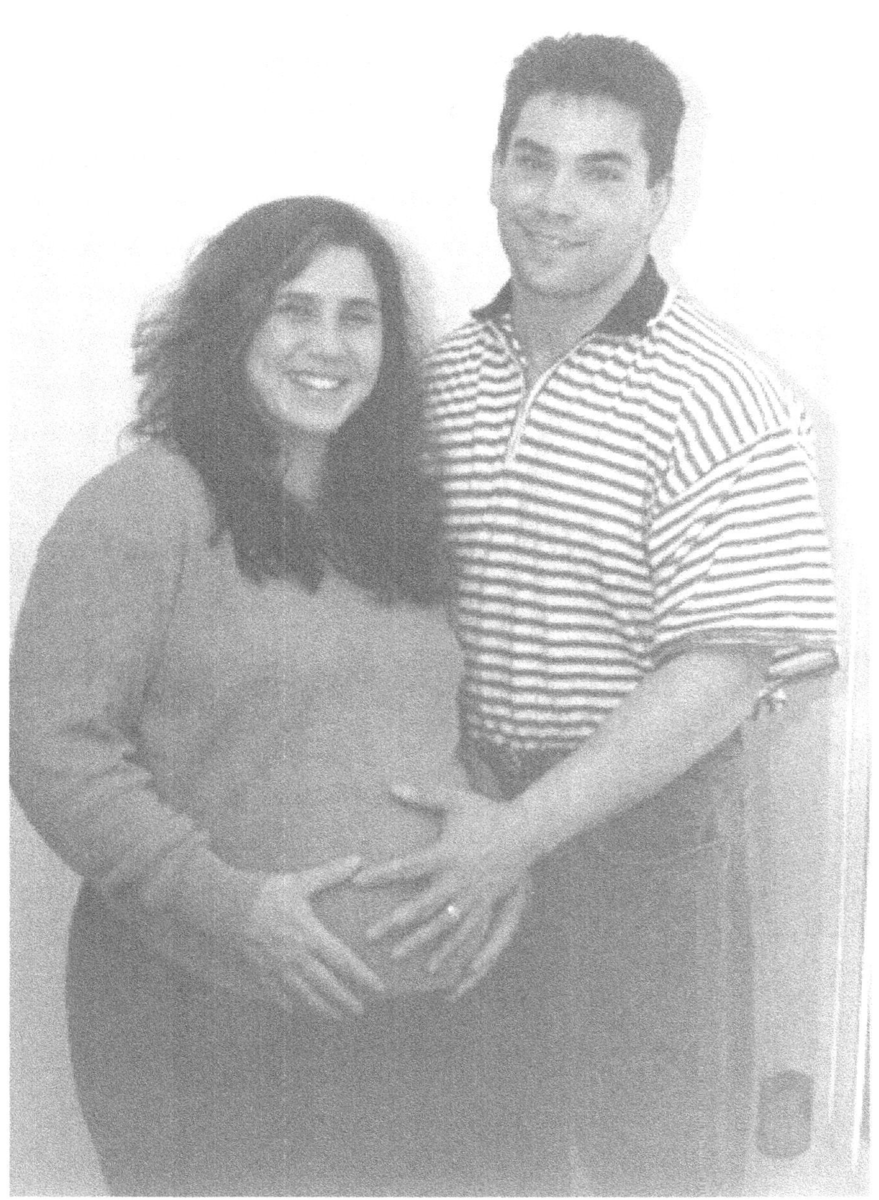

Nine months pregnant and qualifying for the 198-pound weight class.

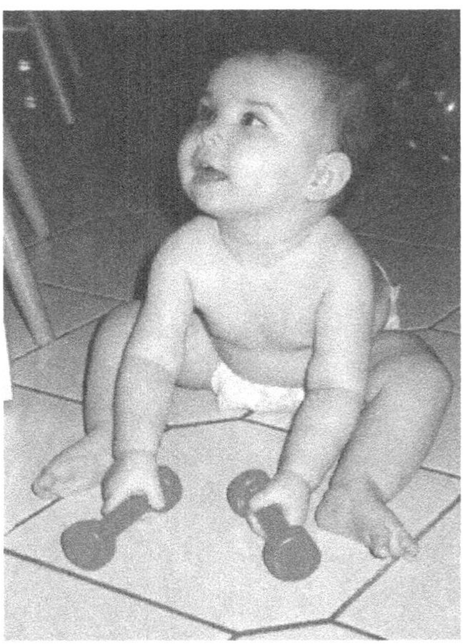

Passing the torch to my little girl, Renée, with her first pair of dumbbells!

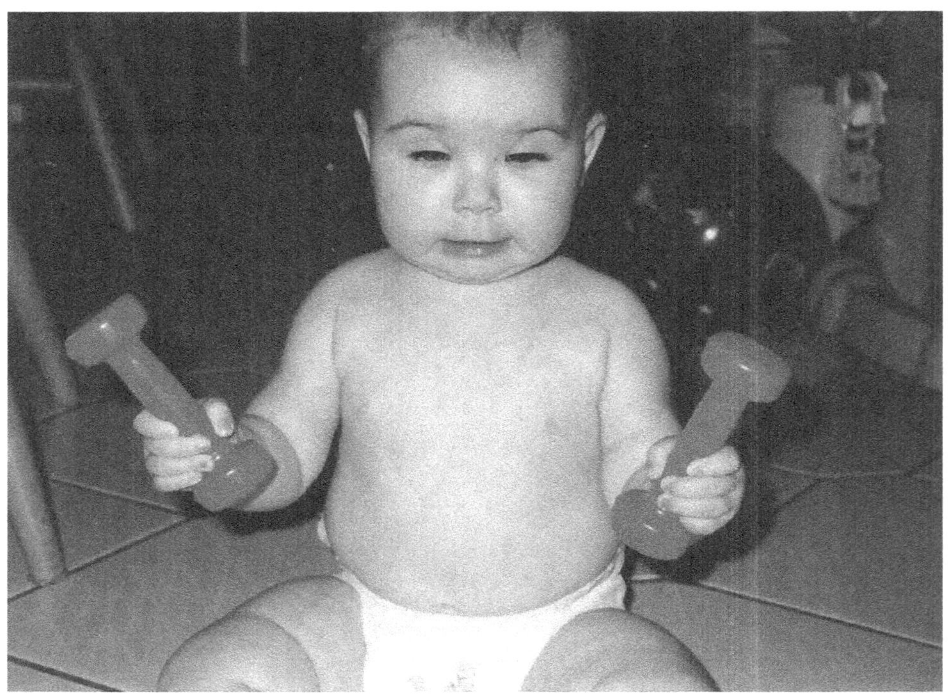

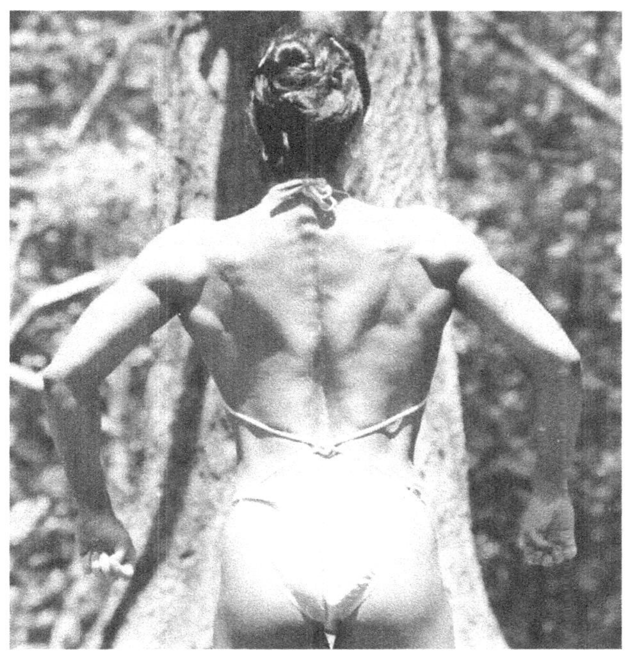

Back muscle development at 20-something.

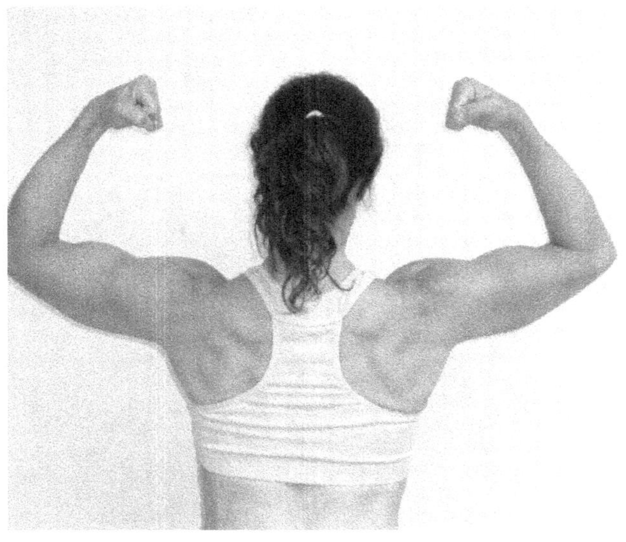

At 40-something.

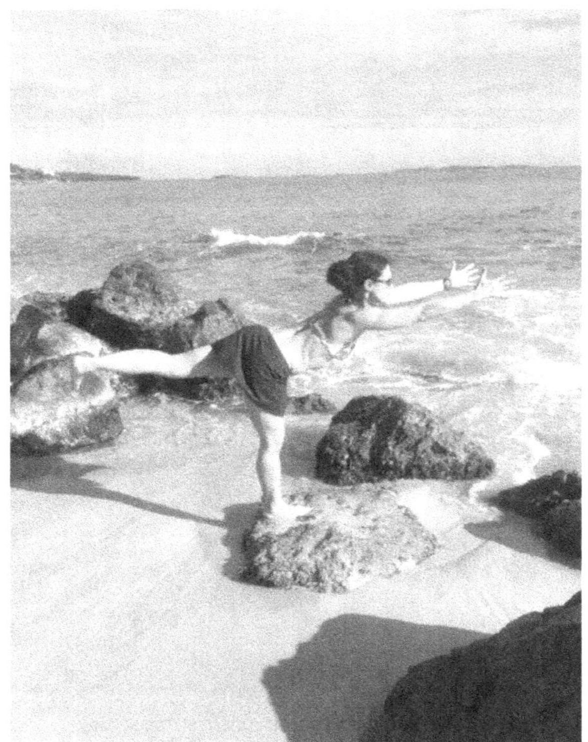

Yoga on the rocks.

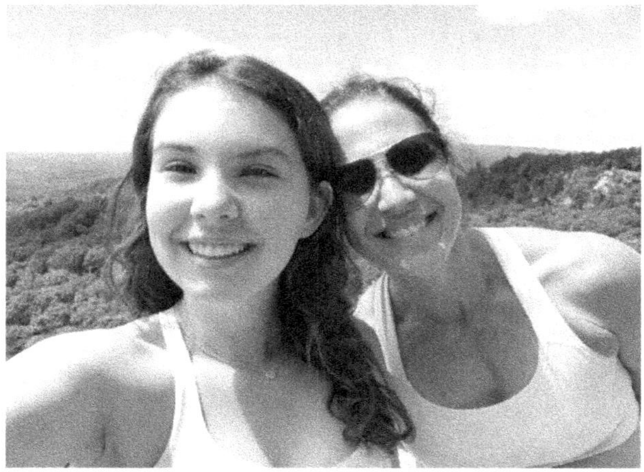

Reaching the summit of the "Lemon Squeeze"
with my favorite female workout partner.

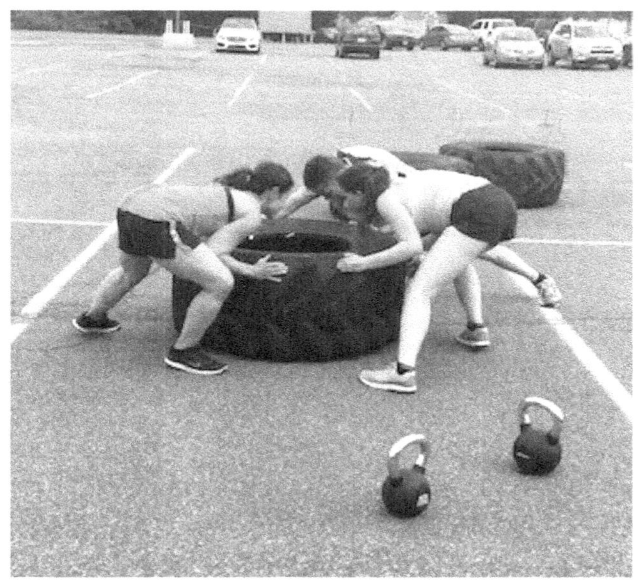

Flipping tires with the family.

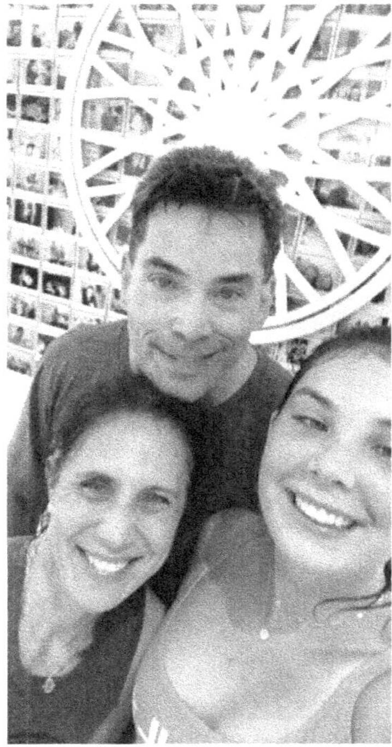

Enjoying a sweaty spin class together.

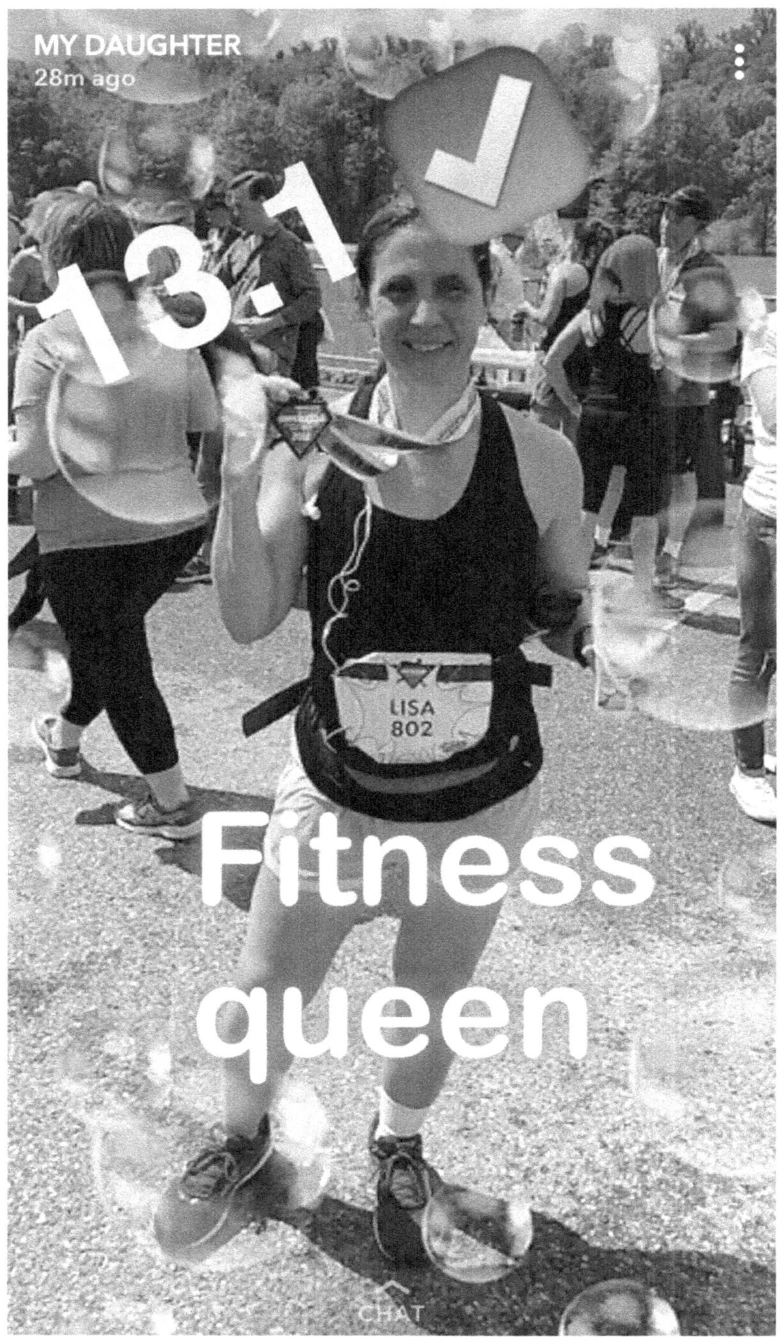

From Renee's SnapChat story after my half-marathon.
Craig and Renee, my two biggest supporters, meet me at the finish line.